The Mayo Clinic Handbook for Happiness

THE
MAYO CLINIC
HANDBOOK FOR
HAPPINESS

A 4-STEP PLAN FOR RESILIENT LIVING

A Companion to *The Mayo Clinic Guide to Stress-Free Living*

Amit Sood, M.D., M.Sc., FACP
Professor of Medicine
Mayo Clinic, Rochester, Minnesota

Da Capo

LIFE
LONG
A Member of the Perseus Books Group

MAYO CLINIC

Managing Editor
Stephanie K. Vaughan

Product Manager
Christopher C. Frye

Editorial Director
Paula M. Marlow Limbeck

Art Directors
Richard (Rick) A. Resnick,
Stewart (Jay) J. Koski

Illustration
Kent McDaniel

Proofreading
Miranda M. Attlesey, Julie M. Maas

Indexer
Steve Rath

Research Librarians
Anthony J. Cook, Amanda K. Golden,
Deirdre A. Herman, Erika A. Riggin

Set in 11-point Palatino Light by Eclipse Publishing Services

Cataloging-in-Publication data for this book is available from the Library of Congress.

First Da Capo Press edition 2015
ISBN: 978-0-7382-1785-7 (paperback)
ISBN: 978-0-7382-1786-4 (e-book)

Published by Da Capo Press
A Member of the Perseus Books Group
www.dacapopress.com

Note: The information in this book is true and complete to the best of our knowledge. This book is intended only as an informative guide for those wishing to know more about health issues. In no way is this book intended to replace, countermand or conflict with the advice given to you by your own physician. The ultimate decision concerning care should be made between you and your doctor. We strongly recommend you follow his or her advice. Information in this book is general and is offered with no guarantees on the part of the author or Da Capo Press. The author and publisher disclaim all liability in connection with the use of this book.

Da Capo Press books are available at special discounts for bulk purchases in the U.S. by corporations, institutions and other organizations. For more information, please contact the Special Markets Department at the Perseus Books Group, 2300 Chestnut Street, Suite 200, Philadelphia, PA, 19103, or call (800) 810-4145, ext. 5000, or email special. markets@perseusbooks.com.

10 9 8 7 6 5 4

To my inspirations — Terry, Judi and Carla
To my loves — Richa, Gauri and Sia
To all of you — striving to create a kinder and happier world
for our planet's children

Contents

Acknowledgments

I don't feel like I wrote this book. This book is written by hundreds of thousands of my patients and learners who have taught me more than I could ever share with them; by tens of thousands of researchers, thinkers and spiritual luminaries whose work has helped me understand the human condition; thousands of colleagues who have helped and supported my work; and by hundreds of friends and loved ones who have together weaved the cushion of comfort and kindness that is my life breath. To each of you, and countless fellow citizens, sung and unsung, who are striving to make the world a better place, I offer my deepest gratitude.

I am grateful to:

Mayo Clinic Complementary and Integrative Medicine program director Dr. Brent A. Bauer for his phenomenal mentorship and support;

Mayo Clinic Complementary and Integrative Medicine program colleagues Drs. Anjali Bhagra, Tony Y. Chon and Jon C. Tilburt; Debbie L. Fuehrer, L.P.C.C.; Barbara S. Thomley; Susanne M. Cutshall, R.N., C.N.S.; Kathryn C. Heroff; and the entire massage therapy, acupuncture and animal-assisted therapy team for their camaraderie and help each step of the way;

Mayo Clinic General Internal Medicine Division leadership, Drs. Paul S. Mueller and William C. Mundell; Rachel L. Pringnitz; Darshan Nagaraju; and Beth A. Borg for their excellent administrative support and direction;

Mayo Clinic Global Business Solutions book team, especially Christopher C. Frye, Stephanie K. Vaughan, Paula M. Marlow Limbeck, and Deirdre A. Herman and her editorial research team, for their phenomenal editing and help;

Perseus Books and Eclipse Publishing teams — Fred Francis, Dan Ambrosio, Mark Corsey and Jane Gebhart — for believing in my work and helping transform this manuscript into an excellent product;

Mayo Clinic Global Business Solutions, especially Dr. Paul J. Limburg, David P. Herbert, Lindsay A. Dingle and Marne J. Gade, for enthusiastic partnership and support;

Mayo Clinic legal and brand team, especially Monica M. Sveen Ziebell and Amy L. Davis, for helping me each step of the way;

Mayo Clinic Department of Medicine team, especially Dr. Morie A. Gertz and Michael (Mike) H. Schryver, for inspiration and support;

Mayo Clinic leadership, specifically Dr. John H. Noseworthy and Jeffrey W. Bolton, for providing the inspiring vision that drives Mayo Clinic each day; and

Every employee at Mayo Clinic for working together to truly live the spirit of our mission: "The best interest of the patient is the only interest to be considered."

I am especially grateful to:

Dr. Kristin S. Vickers Douglas and Debbie L. Fuehrer, L.P.C.C., for their thorough and deeply insightful review;

Dr. David T. Jones for excellent feedback on the brain chapter;

Judi & Terry Paul, and Carla & Russ Paonessa for their generous philanthropic support and mentorship. Terry recently left us for a different world and will be forever in my heart as one of the most inspiring, resilient and kind human beings I ever met.

My heartfelt thanks to:

My parents, Shashi and Sahib Sood, for being the role models of resilience;

My wife's parents, Kusum and Vinod Sood, for loving me as much as my parents;

My brother Kishore and sisters Sandhya and Rajni for their love and unconditional support;

Gauri and Sia, our bundles of joy (and my happiness officers), for being the sweetest teachers any parent could ever dream of; and

My wife Richa, whose faith, love and kindness power each page of this book.

Finally, my gratitude to each patient and learner who has chosen the path of resilience, faith and positivity through life's countless adversities. I hope each one of you finds health, hope, healing and happiness.

Amit Sood, M.D., M.Sc., FACP

@amitsoodmd

Preface

I grew up in a 400-square-foot home in a relatively underprivileged inner-city neighborhood in central India. Lacking any academic interest, I have no doubt that if left to myself, I would be selling tomatoes on a street corner today. But I was extremely fortunate to be born to parents who valued morality and higher education above anything else. With their prodding, guidance, love and occasional spanking, I entered medical school in the fall of 1984.

Tragedy struck my hometown of Bhopal, India, that year. In the middle of the night, a chemical spill killed several thousand people and disabled tens of thousands. Two days later, I showed up at the hospital door. As a novice doctor-in-training, I couldn't do much, but the experience shook my core. In the following few weeks, I witnessed more stories of suffering and survival than most people see in their lifetimes.

The next few years weren't much different. Despite the amazing resilience of the human spirit, poor nutrition and infections — fueled by lack of resources — were widespread, as they still are in many parts of the world. So when I came to the United States in 1995 after 10 years of medical training, I thought I was coming to the Disneyland of the world. I expected every person here would be happy and content, with no stress.

The reality, as you can imagine, didn't match my expectations. I was shocked by the extent of stress and suffering I saw. And it wasn't limited to low-income, inner-city neighborhoods, where I spent the first two years. Everywhere I went, I saw the same pattern. The statistics were staggering. More than 30,000 people committed suicide every year. Nine percent of teenage girls were pregnant. Ten percent of adults had depression. One percent of adults were in prison. And stress was employers' top health care concern. Something was clearly amiss.

I didn't like the labels "hypochondriac" or "time waster" that we stuck on patients experiencing problems such as chronic pain with a normal MRI or angst related to undiagnosed "spells." After all, no one *chooses* to feel stressed or depressed or feel pain.

I faced many unanswered questions. What are these patients experiencing? Why is healing not happening here? This led to deeper questions about the human condition, which led me to wonder, *Why is happiness so elusive?*

The search for answers started me on a journey. I met hundreds of scientists, philosophers and spiritual luminaries, read thousands of research papers and books, and learned from tens of thousands of patients and students over almost two decades. Finding a path to decrease the distress of 21st-century minds became my passion. Slowly, a theme began to take shape.

I realized that most human suffering isn't the human's fault. The design and operation of our brains and minds generate stress. Together, the brain and mind work as a gifted fault-finding machine. The resulting thoughts and emotions we generate around the clock are geared toward securing our safety. Happiness, a secondary goal, is often bypassed.

I learned about the brain's default mode of wandering attention, where we spend half our day, and the mind's inordinate focus on threats and imperfections. I learned that the human mind is intrinsically restless and embarrassingly irrational. I learned how imagination, our most powerful tool, locks us into creating and living countless "what ifs" that trap us into exhausting ruminations, worrying and thinking about catastrophes. I realized that because of our mind's tendency to discount the good, most of life's pleasures stop bringing us pleasure after a while and fail to provide lasting happiness. All of this knowledge helped me come to an important conclusion: The pursuit of gratitude and compassion might provide me with greater happiness than the pursuit of happiness itself.

With good insight into the inner workings of the brain and the mind, I started thinking about the solutions. First, I cleared my head of all the dogmas, beliefs or biases I had held for years. Then, I explored approaches that made sense based on my newfound understanding. I started applying these ideas in clinical practice, with modest results at first. As my understanding, personal practice and communication skills matured, the results became more consistent, sometimes phenomenal. With growing practice and nudges from several patients and colleagues to put it all together in one place, I decided to write this book.

In developing the resiliency program and writing this book, I have balanced seven key aspects that I believe are critical for these programs to be successful.

1. **Scientific.** Several scientific disciplines, particularly neurosciences and psychology, contribute to the program. Further, many research studies have shown that the program as a whole helps decrease stress and anxiety and enhances resilience, quality of life and happiness.

2. **Skills-based.** The program elements distill themselves into a set of skills that you'll be guided to practice in a structured, step-by-step fashion. This book offers solutions.

3. **Simple.** The skills are designed for a busy life, with the focus on simplicity. I believe the simpler the approach, the more likely we are to practice these skills.

4. **Scalable.** You don't have to take two weeks off or seclude yourself in a monthlong silent retreat to master the program. In clinical practice, my colleagues and I teach the core skills in about 60 to 90 minutes.

5. **Structurally sound.** Individual skills integrate and support each other so that the whole becomes greater than the sum of its parts. For example, a program based on compassion alone can lead to compassion fatigue, unless it's strengthened by gratitude, acceptance and meaning. Similarly, forgiveness is a steep mountain to climb without the support of gratitude, compassion and acceptance.

6. **Secular.** The skills aren't biased toward or reflected in the beliefs of one particular faith system. They should appeal equally to people who consider themselves spiritual but not religious, atheist or with a particular faith.

7. **Suited to 21st-century living.** I believe that our minds run much faster and are busier today than those of people living 2,000 or 3,000 years ago. Asking an average person to take an extra hour to meditate may not be practical. The skills can potentially add hours to your day instead of costing time. Further, we've found that the skills presented resonate with the worldview of most people who have taken the training.

This book engages you more directly in the program described in *The Mayo Clinic Guide to Stress-Free Living*. *The Mayo Clinic Guide to Stress-Free Living* is a comprehensive explanation of the philosophical and scientific basis of the program, while this handbook breaks the program down into a structured four-step approach. Mindful of the complexity of this topic and the busyness of your life, this book features a simple program that won't take up much of your time.

Sprinkled throughout this book, you'll see smiley face symbols ☺. Each symbol is followed by a specific practice that may boost your happiness. Consider trying a few of these practices as you read through the book.

This approach is currently taught both in person and online. The in-person course is taught individually or in groups in two basic formats: an abbreviated version called the Stress Management and Resiliency Training (SMART) program, and a longer version called the Transform course. The SMART program has three versions: 60 to 90 minutes, half a day, or a full day. The full Transform course is taught in group sessions over two days; the instructions continue via teleconference and other media for an additional six months. Online programs include a 12-module Resilient Living course with videos, quizzes and practice exercises, shorter programs, quotes, blogs, tweets, and other material. Find more information on these programs at *www.stressfree.org*.

After decades of studying and working with tens of thousands of patients, I believe that this book outlines a potent and practical approach to happiness and well-being that is well-suited to 21st-century living. Clinical practice and many research studies show that this approach decreases stress and anxiety and enhances resilience and happiness. Nothing will make me happier than helping you find greater happiness. I and my colleagues at Mayo Clinic feel privileged and grateful that you have chosen to partner with us on your path to optimal well-being.

I wish you well.

Amit

Prepare Your Mind

Decrease Your Load

Allow me to start with a silly question — actually, a very silly question.

Say I'm flying to Edinburgh on a 10-day vacation. What should I do with my baggage? Choose the best response.

❑ Take no baggage.
❑ Carry the baggage on my head.
❑ Check in my baggage.

I'm sure you chose the third option, "Check in my baggage." Unless I'm competing in one of the "Survivor" contests, "Take no baggage" is not an option. On a family vacation, it's quite the opposite; if you saw our luggage, you'd think we were relocating!

The second choice, "Carry the baggage on my head," also makes no sense. It's dimwitted and impractical.

So what's the lesson here? For starters, how about this thought: When traveling, don't carry your baggage on your head. Check it in.

I suppose that sounds too obvious. Let me offer another perspective, and this time, I'll pose a question. If we don't carry an extra physical load *on* our heads, why do we let our minds carry an extra emotional load *in* our heads?

The mind carries a hefty load of the past and the future that it doesn't need to. Carrying this extra load hurts your mind and causes stress, anxiety and unhappiness. Let's see if we can lighten it, at least for today. Write down the top issues of the past and of the future that are bothering you right now.

Burdens of the past	Burdens of the future

Now imagine that you've put these burdens in a box and stored the box in the attic. You'll collect it tomorrow morning.

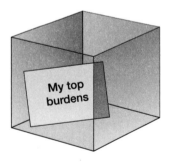

Give yourself a break today. The past before this morning and the future after tonight aren't real. Carry no worries about the world. The ultimate reality is here: you, your seat, your room, this book . . . and this moment. That's it.

Decrease Your Load Even More

I have an idea that will decrease your load even more. I promise I won't be as silly this time.

Based on your life's circumstances, think about what can go wrong in your life in the next hour. Write your thoughts in the box below. Write down only those things that have a good chance of happening.

You may have left the box empty. While life is full of challenges, the stressful events are spread out over a long time span. **Most of the time, the next hour of your life will be OK.**

Do you agree that your day will be more peaceful if you carry only the next hour's load?

Yes ❏   No ❏

If you answered yes, please accept this invitation: Pick only the load of the next one hour while reading this book. These are the things you noted above.

Not the load of yesterday, tomorrow or all of today — only that of the next hour. In fact, you already practice this while driving. Where do you look when you drive your car?

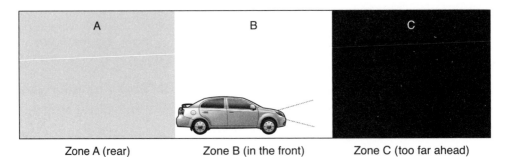

| Zone A (rear) | Zone B (in the front) | Zone C (too far ahead) |

The three zones you can pay attention to as you drive

I'm sure you don't drive constantly looking in the rearview mirror (A) or too far ahead (C). Both are unproductive and dangerous. During most of your drive, you're looking forward, a few hundred feet ahead (B). Granted, occasionally you check the rearview mirror and also may program your GPS at the start of a long drive. But most of your drive happens in this moment. By paying attention to the next few hundred feet, you can cruise through hundreds of miles.

Zone B is on the road. For the mind, that's the next hour.

• • •

Now, perhaps with a lesser load on our minds, let's take a moment to fill our minds with nurturing thoughts. We'll practice my favorite exercise, gratitude meditation.

Take a Moment for Gratitude

Gratitude is acknowledging and appreciating your blessings. Gratitude is your moral memory and represents your thankfulness for every experience. All roads to happiness touch the gratitude milestone.

> 🕊 **Food for Thought:** All roads to happiness touch the gratitude milestone. 🕊

You can be grateful for things, experiences or people. I believe gratitude is most powerful when you apply it to specific people in your life. Let's start by making your gratitude inventory — a list of people in your life you're grateful for.

People in my life I'm grateful for	
My loved ones	
My friends	
My colleagues	
My neighbors	
My teachers	
People who are deceased	
Others (for example, inspiring people, strangers who have been kind to me, pets)	

Do you realize your support network — the people for whom you are grateful — is much bigger than you earlier thought? You're not alone. A whole world out there supports you. On a day when you feel lonely, try to connect with someone in your support network.

> 🕊 **Food for Thought:** You're not alone. A whole world out there supports you. 🕊

Now it's time for the exercise I promised: gratitude meditation. Select five people from your list who you want to remember today. Then carefully read the instructions below.

Once the instructions are clear, close your eyes in a safe, quiet place and practice this meditation. Continue reading after you have completed this exercise.

☺*   Sit in a quiet, comfortable and safe place. Practice deep, slow breathing. Think about the first person you want to be grateful for while taking a deep breath in. Bring this person's smiling face in front of your closed eyes. Make sure you see the face and the smile as distinctly as possible. Now send your silent gratitude (like a mental email) while breathing out. Next, think about the second person. While breathing in, try to visualize that person's smiling face. While breathing out, send your silent gratitude. Repeat this exercise with five people. Relax for a few seconds. When you're ready, open your eyes.

• • •

If you prefer, you can do this exercise with other gifts in your life, instead of people, such as your health, clean air, your home, food, water, the neighborhood you live in, and so on.

---

* ☺ = an exercise that may increase your happiness

How did this brief meditation feel? In the box below, write your feelings in a few words or sentences.

• • •

I feel calm, refreshed and happier when I'm able to decrease my mind's load and think about gratitude. I hope you had a similar experience.

I often wonder something: Why don't we think about gratitude more often? Why do we hold the load of the world in our heads and push away happiness? I think I have some answers — not the perfect answers, but enough to start the conversation. I'd like to share these answers with you next, to help introduce you to your brain and the mind.

Get Your Feet Wet

Your Brain's 2 Modes

With about 90 billion nerve cells that are closely networked and packed in a 3-pound mass the size of a cantaloupe, your brain is much more complex than the Mars rover. But this complexity hides a simple design. Let's unravel the brain's secrets by exploring what keeps it so busy.

Your brain is always doing something, even when you're doing nothing. When it finds the external world interesting, the brain focuses on the world. The brain is generally happy when it's focused, but focus takes effort. The effort is worthwhile when you're entertained or doing something meaningful. But what if the world isn't interesting or meaningful? When it's bored, the brain sulks in its default mode. Its attention wanders, thinking about something other than what you're currently doing or wanting to think about. A wandering mind costs you nothing, but it's very expensive. It causes stress, depression and anxiety, and takes away happiness. If you've ever felt a whirlpool pulling you inside your head, that whirlpool is your brain in its default mode.

All day long, the brain switches between two modes — focused (on something interesting) and default (when your mind wanders or is distracted). Let's look at each of them.

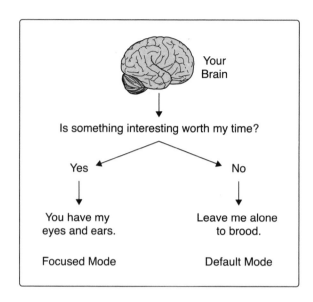

Default Mode? Who, Me? You Must Be Kidding!

While most people recognize their default mode right away, some feel that their attention seldom wanders. That's what I thought, too, until I tested myself. You can take the same test by answering the following questions. Ask yourself:

❏ Have I ever read a book to a child with no idea what I read?
❏ Have I experienced my mind racing in the shower?
❏ Have my thoughts wandered while I was listening to a presentation?
❏ Have I become more forgetful?
❏ Have I woken up recently with thoughts spinning at 100 mph?
❏ Have I fought crazy, distracting ideas during prayer or meditation?
❏ Have I arrived in front of my garage door, wondering how I got there?
❏ Does my spouse or partner complain that I'm often too distracted?

Sound familiar? If you answered yes to any, all these times and more, your brain was in the default mode. The default mode is like the static on your old radio that prevents you from enjoying the crisp music of life.

Now that you recognize your default mode, can you figure out how much of the day you are physically here but mentally somewhere else?

❏ Less than 25 percent
❏ 26 to 50 percent
❏ 51 to 75 percent
❏ More than 75 percent

If you said less than 25 percent, my hat's off to you! I would love to know how you are able to be so focused. But if you selected less than 25 percent, you might want to reconsider — you're probably underestimating how often your mind wanders. That's not me saying this; it's the nerdy scientists. Research shows that our minds wander close to 50 percent of the time or more while we're awake. Right now, as you read this, about 2 to 3 billion people are walking around on our planet with a wandering mind and not much of an idea about what's happening around them.

Sadly, when I talk to people who are stressed, they tell me that most of their day is spent in this mental time travel, as if a hamster were running in their heads. And typically, the hamster isn't having fun running this chase. The following two questions will help explain this.

When are you more likely in the default mode?
❏ On a day when I feel great
❏ On a day when I'm bored
❏ On a day when I feel blah

Research shows that the second and third items are the correct answers. You spend more time inside your head when:

▶ The outside world is boring
▶ You have too many open files — unresolved issues and undone tasks in your life — crammed in your head

What kinds of thoughts do you have when you're in the default mode?

❏ Mostly pleasant
❏ Neutral
❏ Negative

Research shows that most of your thoughts in the default mode are neutral or negative. That's why your brain doesn't have much fun when you leave it alone with itself.

> ✍ **Food for Thought:** Our minds wander close to 50 percent
> of the time we're awake. ☞

The brain creates and continually updates your model of the world with its primary focus on the self (I, me or mine). It weaves stories, makes stuff up by imagining alternative what ifs, and engages in directionless, autobiographical dialogue, pulling superficially related facts from different time periods.

Sounds pretty negative, doesn't it? Please don't get me wrong, though. I don't mean to demonize the default mode. You need healthy default activity. By generating spontaneous thoughts, the default mode connects your past, present and future, helps you understand others from their perspectives, plans your future and hosts your creative insights. It also helps you monitor the external world.

So when does spending time in the default mode become a problem? In two situations:

1. When you spend too much time in the default mode
2. When your spontaneous thoughts constantly dwell on imperfections

You may be wondering about the same thing that I questioned a few years ago: If time in the default mode isn't the happiest, then why is default my brain's preferred parking spot? You'll get the answer in the next section, when I discuss the mind. For now, let's welcome on the stage the second and happier mode of the brain: the focused mode.

The Focused Mode

Imagine if, right at this moment, your best friend from high school or your favorite celebrity walked up to you and shook your hand. What would happen to your attention? Would you forget your stressors for a moment and be totally attentive? If you said yes, it's because your brain is in the focused mode.

Can you recall moments in the past few weeks when you forgot the concerns of everyday life and were so absorbed in something that you totally lost track of time? What were you doing?

❏ Reading a great book
❏ Playing with your child
❏ Watching a gorgeous sunset
❏ Playing tennis or other sport
❏ Solving a client's problem
❏ Visiting a loved one
❏ Enjoying a delicious meal
❏ Praying or meditating

Can you think of other times when you were in this state? Note them below.

These are all focused-mode activities. In the focused mode, you fully attend to the world, appreciating its novelty and meaning. You have few, if any, distractions. You are happier.

While paying attention to something extraordinary is effortless, you can enter a focused mode even when you're paying attention to ordinary objects or people. Three-year-olds spontaneously pay greater attention to ordinary objects because everything is novel to them. But as we get older, the list of things that interest us becomes shorter.

In a typical week, how often are you in the focused mode?
- ❏ Seldom, if ever
- ❏ A couple of times every week
- ❏ Most days
- ❏ Several times every day

Wouldn't it be nice if you could coach your brain to spend more time in the focused mode? Wouldn't it be lovely if five years from now the list of things that interest you is longer than it is today? That's where I hope to take you. I'm sure that on most days, you spend time in the focused mode. I wish to help you substantially increase that time in short, simple steps. The process takes some effort at first, but eventually it becomes effortless.

Let Your Brain Teach Your Brain
Based on what you've learned so far, when are you in the focused mode?

When I'm paying attention to something . . .	❏ Boring	or	❏ Interesting
When I'm paying attention to something . . .	❏ Meaningful	or	❏ Meaningless
When I'm paying attention to something . . .	❏ External	or	❏ In my mind

You most likely selected *interesting, meaningful* and *external*. You are in the focused mode when you're paying attention to something interesting and meaningful, often in the external world. One exception worth mentioning: Intentionally choosing productive, purposeful thoughts also engages your focused mode.

This is an important point that's worth repeating. You're in the focused mode when you're:

▶ Paying attention to something novel and meaningful outside of your mind
▶ Intentionally choosing your thoughts

Between the two, I invite you to initially focus on things outside your mind to train your attention. This is because inner focus — making an effort to intentionally choose your thoughts — often puts you back into the default mode. You may experience this if you struggle with meditation. Most people find an external focus easier to sustain. I will provide details in Section III.

You might say, "I have a lot of stuff I need to think about. How can I just be in the moment?" I totally understand; I'm in the same camp. Instead of being in the moment, I'm asking you to be intentional about how you experience the moment. Let's draw a distinction between two forms of thinking: when you choose your thoughts versus when thinking happens to you. When you choose your thoughts (your thoughts are intentional), they are usually positive and more likely to be productive. But spontaneous thinking stews on imperfections. The former is the focused mode; the latter is the default mode. Here's an example.

> You're sitting in a plane with your husband, Todd, and daughter, Tanya. They both have drifted off to sleep. You start planning Tanya's 10th birthday. It's only a few weeks away. *She really wants a cellphone, but is she old enough? How about a tablet? Maybe an origami book . . .* After a few minutes, you make a mental list. Your thoughts are productive so far. See what happens next. You look at Tanya and remember her friend Anna. Tanya cried this morning because Anna

didn't invite Tanya to her birthday party. Your thoughts start to wander. *Anna's mother didn't return my smile yesterday. I don't care, but Anna's father is Todd's supervisor. What if he fires Todd? How will we pay the mortgage? Should I go back to college and finish my degree? I can't stand statistics. Joining Sherry's jewelry business might ease up some financial pressures. But what if Sherry isn't interested in working with me? How will we put Tanya through college? Can we even afford to have a second child?*

Do you see how the focused mode drifted into the default? You need some default-mode thoughts, but if you don't control them, they'll multiply in your brain like dandelions. I believe we all need to dial down the dialogue in our heads and make our thoughts more positive and productive. I'll share ways to do this in Section III.

● ● ●

Your Brain's 2 Modes: What You've Learned

That's all I have to say about the brain. Forget the details of the different lobes and networks, nerve cells and plexuses, receptors and molecules. Those details may fascinate you, but they'll be distracting. Just knowing about your default and focused modes will take you as far as you need to go in the Resilient Living Program. You can learn more about the brain's two modes in Chapter 1 of *The Mayo Clinic Guide to Stress-Free Living.*

Read each of the following points, reflect on each point for a few moments, and check the box if you understand it well and agree with it.

❑ Your brain has two modes of operation: the focused mode and the default (distracted) mode.
❑ The brain's focused mode processes novel and meaningful information from the world or thinks adaptive, productive thoughts. You're happier in the focused mode.

❑ The brain's default mode processes neutral or negative thoughts and is often experienced as mind wandering. You're not as happy when you spend too much time in the default mode.

❑ People today spend half of their days or more in the default mode, disengaged from or worrying about what's happening in their lives.

One last point: The brain seesaws between the two modes. You can't be distracted and focused at the same time. While this may seem obvious, reflecting on this fact will give you a useful insight: The simplest way to exit unhealthy mind wanderings is to recognize them early and engage your brain with activities that get it into the focused mode.

You're fully alive when you are savoring, are conscious and are conscious that you're conscious. You might have only a few of these moments each day if you spend 80 percent of your time with wandering attention. But if you intentionally engage your brain's focused mode, my hope is that you will be able to literally quadruple your conscious moments.

Is it that simple? Yes, but camping in the focused mode will take some effort. I will need your enthusiastic partnership. I promise to make the journey fun and entertaining.

Your Mind

It's now time to come back to this question: If the focused mode is such a great idea, why do we spend so much time in the default mode? Why do we spend most of our days struggling with our open files — all the unresolved issues in life — increasing our risk of anxiety, depression, attention deficit and maybe even dementia? Let's answer this question by learning the workings of the human mind. In simple terms, think of your brain as your hardware and your mind as its software.

Imagine you're a biological engineer working on a secret experiment to build a new species. What's the most important job you'll assign to that species' mind so that it survives?

❏ Keep the species happy.
❏ Keep the species safe.
❏ Make sure it learns to meditate.
❏ Ensure it sleeps well.

The correct answer is the second one, keep the species safe.

The same holds true for us humans. Your mind's primary job is to keep you and your loved ones safe. Your mind takes stock of information that increases your chance of survival and reproductive success — information that behavioral scientists call salient (valuable). Once safety is secured, the mind starts looking for more interesting stuff.

Which of these items will draw your attention?

In the living room . . .	❏ A snake	or	❏ An ordinary chair
While driving . . .	❏ A white sedan	or	❏ A police car
When hungry . . .	❏ A shoe store sign	or	❏ A pizza shop sign

On the wall . . .	❑ A picture of a convertible	or	❑ A picture of an old house
On the sidewalk . . .	❑ A clown walking	or	❑ A person dressed in ordinary clothes
In the backyard . . .	❑ A robin	or	❑ A bald eagle

You likely selected the snake, police car, pizza sign, convertible, clown and bald eagle. This is because your mind focuses on three things:

▶ Threats (snake and police car)
▶ Pleasure (pizza sign and convertible)
▶ Novelty (clown and bald eagle)

When threat, pleasure and novelty compete, threat is almost always the first thing your mind focuses on. This is a basic human instinct, for obvious reasons. Research shows that we start paying selective attention to threats within the first year of life. Attention to threats helped us survive as a species. The world, however, has changed compared with even a few hundred years ago. Let's see how.

Where Are Our Threats?

How much of your day do you spend totally focused on defending yourself from an actual physical threat?

❑ Less than 10 percent
❑ 11 to 25 percent
❑ 26 to 50 percent
❑ More than 50 percent

I hope you chose less than 10 percent.

What is your best guess about this percentage for a person living 5,000 years ago?

❏ Less than 10 percent
❏ 11 to 25 percent
❏ 26 to 50 percent
❏ More than 50 percent

You may have chosen a higher percentage this time.

Compared with a few thousand years ago, people in most civilized societies today spend much less time guarding their physical safety. For example, in a recent survey, the majority of U.S. women said they aren't afraid to walk alone outside at night.

So where are most of our current threats — in the external world or in the mind? They're in the mind, aren't they?

Our minds are a warehouse of memories and experiences (past hurts and regrets, and future fears) that need resolution. Some of the threats are rational; many are not. Fear is rational when you're in the midst of a physical threat that causes you to FEAR: **f**orget **e**verything **a**nd **r**un. But modern fears often sprout from a different kind of FEAR: **f**alse **e**xpectations **a**ppearing **r**eal. As humorist Mark Twain said, "I have been through some terrible things in my life, some of which actually happened."

The majority of the threats we face today are psychological. Inner battles have replaced outer battles. I fear embarrassing myself, missing a deadline, disappointing someone, or feeling insulted, vulnerable or inadequate. These fears keep our attention locked inside our heads, where we stew (ruminate or worry) about these issues.

Note: Ruminations are repetitive thoughts about the past that may result in sadness, regret, guilt and anxiety. Worries are similar thoughts about the future. In this book, the word *rumination* is meant to represent the negative thoughts related to both the past and the future.

The ruminating mind eventually realizes the futility of its struggles and tries to suppress negative thoughts. But suppressing thoughts is like tightening a spring: the tighter it gets, the stronger it recoils. Research shows that thought suppression leads to more thoughts about the same issue. Your extraordinary imagination, which can think of and catastrophize about all kinds of possibilities, doesn't help. Your brain experiences everything you imagine as if it has already happened. Remembering a person activates the same nerve cells in the brain that are activated by seeing the person's picture.

> 🕊 **Food for Thought:** Your brain experiences everything you imagine
> as if it has already happened. 🕊

The memory of a hurt, rumination about it, unsuccessful attempts at thought suppression and our tendency to catastrophize all lead to attention-drawing pools in the mind that I like to call attention black holes.

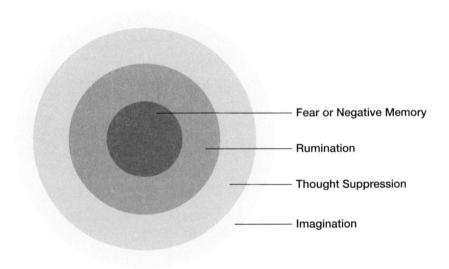

The anatomy of an attention black hole: A kernel of fear or negative memory is surrounded by layers of thoughts created by the mind — an avoidant response that in effect increases attention to the fear or negative memory — and imagination.

Note: The mind also carries pleasant memories and exciting anticipation of happy future events. Instinctively, however, we are more drawn to imperfections than we are to positive events. For this reason and for the sake of simplicity, I will focus primarily on attention black holes.

These black holes could be related to work pressures, relationship insecurity, economic struggles, a past hurt or a medical concern. They take your attention away from the splendor of the world and into mind wandering and mental time travel. The process drains energy, feeds on itself and leads to stress.

Here's an example. Let's say your doctor leaves this voice mail for you at 4:30 p.m. today: "Bob, call me ASAP. I need to tell you about your test results." You check your messages at 9 p.m. and call back, but nobody answers the phone. Will you fear the worst, worry through the night and then try to suppress your worries so you can get some sleep? If you said yes, you were caught in a black hole.

Do you have any black holes related to your personal or professional life that draw your attention? Write them in the space below.

	Past	Future
Personal (family, relationships, health, home and so on)		
Professional		

Many of us carry multiple black holes that draw our attention toward the imperfections of the past and the future and away from the here and now.

In addition to the black holes, we also carry numerous open files in our heads. The fast pace of life, rapidly changing technologies and a phenomenal number

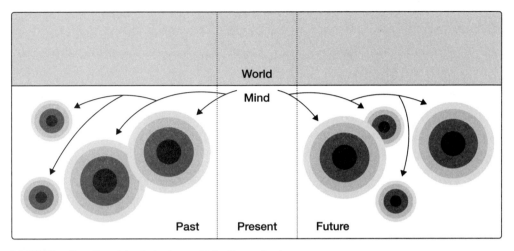

Multiple attention black holes within the mind

of choices force our minds to drive in the left lane all day. Most people I meet pay dozens of bills every month and have to memorize as many or more user IDs and passwords. The result of the fast pace and open files is that you struggle to quiet your train of thoughts as the hamster races uncontrollably. The world starts seeming dull.

The constant company of hurts, regrets, fears and open files increases the time you spend in the survival mode. Billions of us live in this state. I think just one person living in this mode is too many.

• • •

Your Mind: What You've Learned

Read each of the following points, reflect on each point for a few moments and check the box next to it if you agree and understand it well.

❏ Our attention can be drawn toward the world, the mind or both.
❏ Attention depends on motivation.
❏ Threat serves as the primary motivator. Pleasure and novelty also motivate, but they are weaker than threat.

- ❏ The majority of modern threats are inner emotional battles.
- ❏ On most days, the external world doesn't send us many serious threats or extraordinary pleasures.
- ❏ Our inner emotional battles are stockpiled as attention black holes.
- ❏ Attention black holes cause our attention to be effortlessly drawn into the mind.
- ❏ In the mind, attention gets stuck with the imperfections of the past and the future, and all of the open files.
- ❏ We start living our lives mostly in our minds.
- ❏ Surrounded by hurts, regrets, fears and open files, we bypass happiness and, instead, live an unfulfilled life.

At the end of the previous section, I blamed the mind for forcing us into the default mode. I'll make one amendment to this. The mind only does the job assigned to it, which is to protect us. A lot of our stress relates to instincts that helped us survive and made us the dominant species. Stress becomes ingrained in the way our brains and minds instinctively operate.

You may ask, *Why are some of us more stressed, depressed or anxious than others?* Perhaps our brains came wired that way, are biologically predisposed, or we weren't treated kindly as children or as adults, and we're unable to purge the negative energy.

The one lesson I have learned is this: Be kind to anyone experiencing stress — including yourself.

● ● ●

We haven't yet had a serious discussion about stress or resilience. Let's start with a few thoughts on happiness as a first step and then move to stress.

Happiness

Look around you and notice who seems really happy in this world. It's little kids. Every child comes wired with a magical ability to find joy in the mundane. The happiest person I know is our 3-year-old daughter, Sia. A Tootsie Roll is enough to get her excited. What makes children so naturally happy? Four attributes come to mind. Check the ones you agree with.

- ❏ Children get happy with little things.
- ❏ They don't dwell on life's challenges.
- ❏ They actively seek the novel and the pleasant.
- ❏ They don't try to improve others.

I had all these gifts many years ago. But then life happened. My mind got busy with all of its open files. I didn't realize that the party was happening outside my head, not inside. My days became filled with finding faults and avoiding fear, rather than fulfilling passion. As the years rolled by, I began bypassing happiness.

Happiness is the state of experiencing positive emotions. Happiness depends on two key ingredients: feeling safe and feeling worthy. When you feel physically or emotionally unsafe or have low self-worth, no material gain can provide lasting happiness. Once you feel safe and worthy, pleasant immersive experiences, creative work, meaningful pursuits and altruistic thoughts and actions all enhance happiness.

Research shows that up to 50 percent of our happiness depends on our conscious choices that, with time, become enduring habits. Most material gains, on the other hand, provide happiness only for a short time because of our tendency to quickly discount the good and rearrange our expectations. Remember your last promotion. How long did the joy of the promotion last? Most people say a few days at most. Now imagine being passed over for promotion. How long does the frustration of being passed over last? It lasts for a long time, doesn't it? Our tendency to discount the good and inflate the bad pushes away happiness. But we can learn from the truly happy people in our society — children and the elderly.

The happiest people in our society are children and the elderly. Children's happiness depends on feeling loved, having pleasant immersive experiences and not spending time with negative ruminations. The elderly — particularly those who develop wisdom as they age — entertain a more mature perspective, have lower expectations, seek a higher meaning that has elements of altruism and focus on savoring rather than catastrophizing. By learning the lessons of innocence from children and wisdom from the elderly, we can internalize the happiness habit.

Happiness is a habit. Some of us are born with it; others have to choose it. Unfortunately, many people don't realize they have to make the choice. Or if they do realize it, they don't find a good path. A lot of your happiness is up to you and your choices. Several situations in life, such as the loss of a loved one, a health crisis or financial insecurity, are bound to make you unhappy. But in many situations, you have a choice. If you are beside yourself because of spilled milk on the dining table, a leaky faucet or weak coffee, then you aren't prioritizing happiness.

A healthy insight into life's challenges is a good first step toward making happiness a priority.

Let me ask you: In which of the following ways is your life presently challenged? Check all that apply.

❑ Relationships
❑ Health
❑ Finances
❑ Work
❑ Other _____
❑ Other _____

Do you think your challenges are likely to increase, decrease, go away or stay the same over the next five years? Mark your answers in the space provided on the next page.

	Increase	Decrease	Go away	Stay the same
Relationships	❏	❏	❏	❏
Health	❏	❏	❏	❏
Finances	❏	❏	❏	❏
Work	❏	❏	❏	❏
Other _____	❏	❏	❏	❏
Other _____	❏	❏	❏	❏

Did you check "Go away" for any of the options? In most situations, stressors will increase, decrease or stay about the same. This understanding is the first step to prioritizing happiness.

Do not postpone happiness, waiting for a day when life will be perfect and all of your stressors will disappear. If you wait because you are too busy or stressed, you might wait a lifetime. Your opportunity to live as well as you can is in this very moment. If you let go of this opportunity, you might come back to it, maybe a decade later. You will lose precious time in the process.

You'll always have some excuse. I myself have never had a day when my boat was fully secure in the harbor, the water was deep blue, the winds were quiet, and the sun was bright and shining in the sky. The wait for such a day will be very long. So I need to admit the reality and find fulfillment in the present moment, accepting all its imperfections. I need to awaken the child and the sage within me today.

The important next question is, What gets in the way of happiness?

Stress

You push happiness away when you feel too much stress. Stress is your struggle with what is. Stress starts with not having what you want or not wanting what you have. If you like what you have and love those who belong to you, you'll have minimal stress.

Stressors and Stress

Knowing the difference between stressors and stress is useful. Stressors are the triggers (events, people and so on); stress is how you view the nuisance stressors can or have caused you. Perception has several components: how bad the threat is, how well you can respond to it, if your response will take away the threat, and what it all means to you. You often can't remove stressors, but you can decrease the stress they cause by changing how you view them.

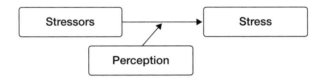

Let's look at the effect of your perception in this example. In the list below, make note of everything in the world that makes you happy. Don't check any of the boxes yet.

1. _____ ❏

2. _____ ❏

3. _____ ❏

4. _____ ❏

5. _____ ❏

6. _____ ❏

7. _____ ❏

8. _____ ❏

Now go back and check those items that were or are a source of stress.

Do you realize that your sources of stress and joy are the same?

Welcome to the world that has two names: Joyville and Stressville. Stress and opportunity are inseparable. The face of a stressor has the body of an opportunity. Your challenges are also your playground, your life's breath. You can't wish them away.

Now that you recognize that stressors will lurk forever in your backyard, let's develop a healthier approach to coping with them. We'll first classify your stressors into three groups: personal, work-related and others. We'll then evaluate why some stressors are a source of happiness, while others feel like a heavy load.

Let's start by listing your stressors.

Personal stressors (family, home, relationships, health)	
Work-related stressors	
Others	

Why Some Stressors Become Stressful

Stressors and related stress come in three flavors: good, bad and ugly.

Good	We welcome this stress.	Having a baby, vacation, promotion or party; getting married
Bad	We are overwhelmed by this stress.	Excessive workload, financial loss, illness in the family, argument with spouse, children squabbling with each other
Ugly	We want to avoid hurtful or catastrophic events at all cost.	Diagnosis of terminal cancer, unexpected divorce, philandering spouse, loss of a loved one

Our goal is to keep the good stress, convert the bad stress into the good stress and be prepared for the ugly stress, while hoping it never comes. Three things that change the good stress into bad or ugly stress are:

1. Demand-resource imbalance
2. Lack of control
3. Lack of meaning

1. Demand-resource imbalance

When the demands placed on you exceed your capacity to meet them, you feel stressed. Have you ever felt overwhelmed because you had too much to do in too little time? How often, where and when does this happen to you?

How often?		Where?	
Every day	❏	At work	❏
Several times a week	❏	At home	❏
A few times a month	❏	Other places	❏
Rarely	❏	**When?**	
		Weekdays	❏
		Weekends	❏

Notice the times and places where you perceive a demand-resource imbalance. In the box below, identify the stressors related to demand-resource imbalance and think of ways you can overcome them. For example, can you delegate, be more efficient or skip the activity altogether?

Stressor*	Ideas to overcome demand-resource imbalance

*A stressor that is related to demand-resource imbalance can also be a stressor because of lack of control or lack of meaning.

2. Lack of control

Control is power. Control gives you freedom to choose. Lack of control leads to fear. You may wonder when the next shoe will drop and how heavy it will be. When you're in control, you feel relaxed and optimistic and are more willing to help others.

Have you ever felt treated like a doormat? Have you felt your preferences were purposefully ignored? How often does that happen, where and when?

How often?		**Where?**	
Every day	❏	At work	❏
Several times a week	❏	At home	❏
A few times a month	❏	Other places	❏
Rarely	❏	**When?**	
		Weekdays	❏
		Weekends	❏

Notice the times and places where you feel a lack of control. In the box below, identify the stressors related to lack of control and think of ways you can overcome them. For example, can you find aspects in your experience that are still in your control? What about spending less time with people who don't respect you? Asserting yourself more effectively? Or accepting that you can't change some things?

Stressor*	Ideas to overcome lack of control

*A stressor that is related to lack of control can also be a stressor because of demand-resource imbalance or lack of meaning.

3. Lack of meaning

We are a meaning-seeking species. You do what you do because you find it meaningful. Being able to find meaning and something positive amid adversity is the hallmark of resilience.

Each year, approximately 130 million babies are born. Despite sleepless nights, fatigue and pain, most moms don't see childbirth as suffering. They see the precious positive meaning in the birth of a beautiful baby. The pain of a kidney stone, however, always brings suffering because it lacks a positive meaning.

Are there times you lose sense of meaning in your work? Do you experience adversity for which you can't find any meaning? How often does that happen to you and where? Make note of them on the next page.

How often?		Where?	
Every day	❏	At work	❏
Several times a week	❏	At home	❏
A few times a month	❏	Other places	❏
Rarely	❏	**When?**	
		Weekdays	❏
		Weekends	❏

🕊 **Food for Thought:** A stressor becomes stressful when it is greater than your capacity to handle it, isn't within your control or doesn't have adequate meaning. 🕊

Notice the times and places where you perceive a lack of meaning. In the box below, identify your stressors related to lack of meaning and think of ways you can overcome them. For example, can you look at your responsibilities from the perspective of others whom you are helping? Decrease negative meaning by recognizing that most of your fears won't come true? Find positive meaning by seeing how adversity has helped you? Find meaning in how your adverse situation prevented something worse?

Stressor*	Ideas to overcome lack of meaning

*A stressor that is related to lack of meaning can also be a stressor because of demand-resource imbalance or lack of control.

What is, was or might be often isn't negotiable, but you can always soften your struggle. Here's one logical way to approach stress.

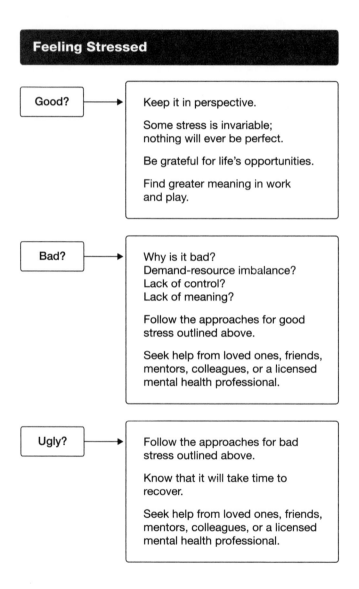

Feeling Stressed

Good? → Keep it in perspective.

Some stress is invariable; nothing will ever be perfect.

Be grateful for life's opportunities.

Find greater meaning in work and play.

Bad? → Why is it bad?
Demand-resource imbalance?
Lack of control?
Lack of meaning?

Follow the approaches for good stress outlined above.

Seek help from loved ones, friends, mentors, colleagues, or a licensed mental health professional.

Ugly? → Follow the approaches for bad stress outlined above.

Know that it will take time to recover.

Seek help from loved ones, friends, mentors, colleagues, or a licensed mental health professional.

Before we wrap up our discussion on stress, I would like to offer one additional perspective.

How Do You See Your Stressors?

How do you describe your stressors? Check all that apply.

- ❏ Punishment
- ❏ Defeat
- ❏ Loss
- ❏ Enemy
- ❏ Challenge
- ❏ Value
- ❏ Opportunity
- ❏ Growth

When you see stressors as punishment, defeat or loss, or as the enemy, you add layers of emotional suffering. Such stressors form the origin for negative memories that keep you away from the wonders of life. By viewing stressors as value, an opportunity, a challenge or growth, you harness them to advance in life. If you get short of breath after climbing 10 stairs, it shows you need to get more physical activity. Likewise, a feeling of stress might be a sign that you need to become more resilient or bring your life to a greater balance.

In reality, most stressors can prompt you toward growth. Think about your past challenges. Did anything good come out of them? Which of the following resulted from your challenges?

- ❏ Helped me connect better with relatives or friends
- ❏ Gave me an opportunity to learn
- ❏ Helped me develop a broader outlook toward life
- ❏ Connected me with my spirituality
- ❏ Helped me appreciate my blessings
- ❏ Made me more grateful for what I have
- ❏ Tested my resilience and ultimately made me stronger
- ❏ Other _____
- ❏ Other _____

You can choose to see most of your stresses as a source of growth. Your life is a beautiful mosaic with multiple colors. All the colors have their place. Absolute good is an illusion. Everything is a combination of good and bad. What feels bad today may be good tomorrow and vice versa. See how the colors fit together.

Try to embrace others' imperfections to the extent that you can. This step is the first and most essential toward their transformation — and your own.

Like an appetizing menu, many (but not all) things in life are here for the asking. Do not place your request based on what you see on others' tables. Create your own plate based on your preferences, appetite and palate. Make sure you keep enough servings of love and peace, not just as dessert at the end of the dinner, but also part of the main course.

You may not have much control over your stressors, but how you view them depends entirely on you. Your perceptions determine how you respond to the disruptions.

> ✐ **Food for Thought:** Three tools can convert a bad stressor into a good stressor: securing balance between demand and resources, cultivating a sense of control, and finding meaning in work and in play. Taking these steps will make you happier and resilient. ☞

Resilience

Think about three or more people you know whose spirits can't be put down by any adversity. They bounce back from whatever life throws at them. Maybe your grandma or great-grandma provided the solid anchor to your family. Or your dad has the fortitude to withstand any storm. I'm sure there are many others you admire. Think about what contributes to their strength.

Then, in the space provided below, list the people you're thinking of to the left in the table. To the right of each name, list what you consider to be that person's source(s) of strength.

Person	Source(s) of strength

The people you listed are resilient. Resilience is your ability to prevent, withstand and bounce back from adversity. It helps you bend but not break. Research shows that resilience is related to taking on a challenge rather than getting overwhelmed, having a sense of control and finding meaning in what you are doing. Resilience has four domains: physical, cognitive, emotional and spiritual.

> ✒ **Food for Thought:** Resilience has four domains.
> Physical resilience is maintaining the best possible health.
> Cognitive resilience is maintaining focus amid stress.
> Emotional resilience is approaching life's challenges with a realistic,
> flexible and balanced disposition, and having good control over your
> emotions. Spiritual resilience is finding an anchor in higher meaning
> and a selfless perspective. ☞

Physical resilience is being strong and healthy, and recovering quickly from illness or injury. An active lifestyle, healthy eating, adequate sleep, nurturing relationships, optimal self-care, timely medical and preventive care, and a good handle on stress all contribute to physical resilience.

Cognitive resilience is your ability to maintain focus in the midst of stress. Focus, insight and decision-making suffer during excessive stress. Let's take a simple example: losing your car keys on a Monday morning. It's 7:30 a.m. and you have to be at work by 8 a.m. After a 10-minute search, you still can't find your keys. What happens to your attention at that time? Aren't you frazzled, hoping someone will come and help? Time pressures lessen the quality of your attention. My keys could be right in front of me, but I can't see them. (I have heard it called male-pattern blindness!)

Cognitive resilience prevents loss of focus. It can sometimes be lifesaving, as it was when Capt. Chesley "Sully" Sullenberger landed US Airways Flight 1549 on the surface of the Hudson River after the plane was disabled by a flock of Canada geese.

Attention training enhances cognitive resilience — an aspect we will turn to in Section III.

Emotional resilience is the experiencing of positive emotions and recovering quickly from negative emotions. Helen Keller lost her vision and hearing when she was barely 2 years old. She went on to write 12 books and was among the most admired people of the 20th century. She didn't withdraw from life or sulk in a dark basement. She dealt with adversity and tried to make the best of her limitations — the very definition of emotional resilience — by approaching rather than withdrawing from challenges.

Spiritual resilience is the ability to maintain a higher meaning and selfless perspective despite facing adversity and disappointments. When he came out of prison after 27 years, Nelson Mandela was brimming with forgiveness and compassion, rather than consumed by thoughts of revenge and violence. Mahatma Gandhi remained anchored in nonviolence, risking his life many times. They are examples of spiritual resilience. When life throws an obstacle in your path, spiritual resilience helps you recover and get back on the highway.

Note all of the people you consider resilient and in which domains you find them resilient.

Person	Physical	Cognitive	Emotional	Spiritual
	❑	❑	❑	❑
	❑	❑	❑	❑
	❑	❑	❑	❑
	❑	❑	❑	❑
	❑	❑	❑	❑
	❑	❑	❑	❑
	❑	❑	❑	❑

With inspiration from these people and from the ideas we've discussed, can you think of ways to increase your resilience? Write your ideas on the next page.

I can increase my:
Physical resilience by . . .
Cognitive resilience by . . .
Emotional resilience by . . .
Spiritual resilience by . . .

The path to resilience and happiness in this program has two steps:

1. Self-discovery
2. Self-transformation

Self-discovery involves discovering your stressors, understanding the concepts of human stress, resilience and happiness, and knowing the workings of your brain and the mind. We have already made some progress on these topics. Next we'll pursue the second step in the program: Becoming happier and more resilient by developing intentional and strong attention and emotional (and spiritual) resilience. Intentional attention will dial down the voice in your head and offer you greater power to choose your thoughts, words and actions. Emotional resilience will help you align your thoughts and feelings with timeless principles that are essential for your success and key to lasting happiness.

Let's take the plunge and learn these skills.

Take the Plunge

Introducing the 4-Step, 10-Week Program

In four simple steps, this 10-week program is designed to provide you a structured, scientific and practical approach to integrate its principles into your life. The steps follow a logical, thoughtful sequence that has been tested and found to be useful in multiple research studies.

The First Step: Train Your Attention

Attention is the gateway into your mind. Trained attention empowers you to better regulate what you think and perceive. For most of us, such attention isn't innate and needs to be cultivated. How strong do you think your attention is?

❑	❑	❑	❑	❑
1	2	3	4	5
Weak	OK	Strong	Very strong	As good as it can be

If you think you have perfect attention, try to answer these questions:

Do I sometimes forget where I parked my car?

Do I experience work-related ruminations after I get home?

Do I have the urge to check emails while spending time with my family?

Have I consumed an entire meal without experiencing most of it?

Have I made quick judgment about someone, only to regret it later?

Have I experienced mind-wandering during prayer or meditation?

Do I struggle with remembering people's names?

If you answered yes to any of the above, training your attention might help.

Attention training offers a practical, time-efficient approach to sprinkle multiple moments of authentic, undistracted presence in your world. Trained attention pulls you out of your head into your life. The specific practices I'll offer are carefully chosen so that they not only train your attention but also are enjoyable. I see them as adding chocolate powder to your glass of milk. Within a few weeks, you'll start looking forward to each practice. Further, the practice won't cost you any extra time; instead it might save you several hours every day by decreasing unhelpful ruminations.

The Second Step: Cultivate Emotional Resilience

Our minds are storehouses of rapid judgments, instincts and reflexive behaviors geared toward safety and survival. Sometimes these quick responses are helpful. But more commonly, they lead us astray. Have you ever overreacted to what later seemed like a trivial issue? If you answered yes, you have room to grow in self-awareness and self-control, and in attuning yourself with others' feelings. All of these skills can be enhanced by increasing your emotional resilience.

Emotionally resilient people experience positive emotions on most days, preserve emotional stability through adversity and recover positive emotions relatively quickly after facing adversity. They maintain a realistic, flexible and balanced disposition and generally approach — rather than withdraw from — life's challenges. They find life meaningful, have a sense of control and, when needed, are OK with letting go of control.

Emotional resilience swaps your instinctive prejudices and biases with five core principles: gratitude, compassion, acceptance, meaning and forgiveness. Gratitude reminds you of how blessed you are, even amid adversity. Compassion helps you recognize and heal others' pain and suffering. Acceptance allows you to creatively work with what is and be open to possibilities. Meaning inspires you to make the world a better place and find greater joy in what you do. Forgiveness recognizes imperfections among all of us and empowers you to free yourself by deliberately letting go of the hurts.

Each principle, intentionally practiced, provides a nurturing alternative to the mind so that it stops stewing in negativity. Such a mind becomes free of fear and unhealthy wants. A mind so freed fosters the most important aspect of your life — your relationships.

The Third Step: Start a Mind-Body Practice

As you advance in this journey, you reach a point where you are no longer satisfied with sampling life at its surface. You want to know and experience life in greater depth. A personal mind-body practice that resonates with your beliefs and is practical for you then becomes essential for your growth.

The specific practice is a combination of trained attention and emotional resilience, often mixed with elements that reflect your worldview. Meditation and prayer are the two most well-known mind-body practices. However, no matter the practice you choose, the goal is the same — to become a calmer, happier, stronger and kinder human being.

The Fourth Step: Pick Healthy Habits

We do most of our routine activities out of habit. You brush your teeth, take a shower, drink coffee in the morning, drive to work, eat popcorn while watching TV — all of these habits require minimal conscious effort. These habits form after you repeat a conscious behavior over and over, until it gets programmed in your brain. Healthy habits help your health; unhealthy habits hurt your health. There's a good chance you have an unhealthy habit you wish to change. There's also a good chance you have tried to change this habit (by losing weight, exercising, quitting smoking, cutting down on alcohol) but have not consistently succeeded.

Why is it that while most of us know the right thing to do, it's so difficult to resist that fat- and sugar-laden doughnut? The reason is simple — resisting our innate urges (that is, self-control) takes effort. Effort consumes energy. That energy comes from a single bucket of vitality (or will power). With chronic stress, the bucket is leaky and loses vitality. My humble hope is that through the Resilient Living Program, you will enhance your vitality and thus improve your ability to pick one healthy habit. I have observed this change countless times among our course participants. Before we complete our journey together through this book, I'll invite you to make one positive change in your life, so that this program improves your physical health, in addition to emotional and mental health.

Let's now take the first step in the 10-week Resilient Living Program: training your attention.

The First Step: Train Your Attention

Weeks 1–2: Joyful Attention and Kind Attention

Life is a series of experiences. Let's analyze a simple experience, looking at the pen in the picture below.

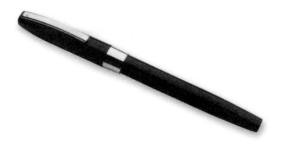

I'm sure you've seen hundreds of pens like this one. Your brain and mind experience the pen in two simple steps: attention and interpretation.

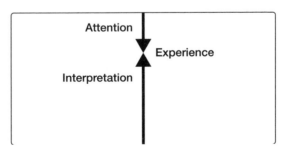

Attention meets interpretation to create an experience.

Attention brings information about the pen into your brain. Since you have memory of how a pen looks, your brain launches a quick interpretation. Where attention and interpretation meet, you have an experience: You figure out that this is a pen.

Once you determine that this is an ordinary pen, your attention finds no reason to continue looking at it. You move on to the next thing. This moving on is necessary, helpful and efficient. But there is one problem: You move on too quickly.

As we get older, we store countless memories in our brains that block deeper attention. Once loaded with these interpretations, we prematurely stop paying attention to the world because we already know everything. Why do we need to look at the ordinary? We still see the pen, but not this very pen. In this state, we skim through life. We miss paying attention to life's most important and enjoyable aspects — our loved ones. We forget that joy is in the details, the particulars, the specifics — and not in the biased generalizations. Life's happiest moments and lasting memories need immersive experience.

How can you get such immersive experience? With deeper attention and delayed interpretations. Attention training is developing the deeper attention.

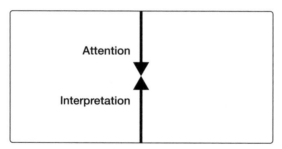

Attention and interpretation within the brain. Note that the attention arrow is now longer than in the previous illustration.

🪶 **Food for Thought:** Deeper attention and delayed interpretations lead to an immersive experience and lasting memories. 🖋

Here, you might ask: *Most of my days are ordinary. I'm neither running away from mammoths nor having a date with my favorite celebrity. How can I then focus on this boring world?*

I see why you ask this question. Once you're familiar with the world, including people around you, it stops holding your attention. Realize that the world won't change for you. But with training, you can cultivate a deeper attention that no longer depends on threat or pleasure. It is guided by novelty. You discovered novelty when you were a child, but your ability to do this fades as you age. Attention training wakes up the child in you who found the world novel and fascinating, and a place to have fun.

> ✐ **Food for Thought:** Attention training wakes up the child in you who found the world novel and fascinating, and a place to have fun. ✐

Based on what you've learned so far, answer this question: How would you describe trained attention? Mark your answers below.

❑ Predominantly directed toward the world	or	❑ Internal toward the mind
❑ Focused on threat	or	❑ Focused on novelty
❑ Quick and judgmental	or	❑ Delayed judgment

I'm sure you got the right answers:

▶ Predominantly directed toward the world
▶ Focused on novelty
▶ Delayed judgment

We will use these three key attributes to train our attention, the next step. The two broad approaches to attention training are:

1. **Joyful attention.** Delaying judgment and paying attention to novelty.
2. **Kind attention.** Attending with compassion and acceptance.

Week 1: Joyful Attention

Joyful attention is:

▶ Focused
▶ Relaxed
▶ Compassionate
▶ Nonjudgmental
▶ Sustained
▶ Deep
▶ Intentional

Joyful attention engages the focused mode of the brain and gently redirects your mind to find greater novelty.

In this section, I'll share three core joyful attention skills, suggest ideas for additional practice and integrate the approach into a structured program. Our goal is to cultivate a discipline that allows us to sprinkle several moments of joyful attention throughout the day.

Core Joyful Attention Skills: Three Exercises

Exercise 1: Wake Up With Gratitude and in the Moment

After you wake up in the morning, how long does it take for your mind to start wandering?

❑ Less than five seconds
❑ A few minutes
❑ More than 15 minutes
❑ Doesn't happen to me

The most common answer is "less than five seconds." Most people are in the focused mode for only a few seconds after they wake up and, very quickly, their minds wander. I have asked thousands of people about the first thoughts that greet them in the morning. See their top two answers on the next page.

1. What should I do today?
2. What should I dread today?

I call these thoughts the "do-dread duo." In this state, we wake up feeling insecure.

Then, many of us do one more activity that traps us in the mind: check email. The telegraphic messages in emails create a fresh set of open files that keep us busy in our heads, just when we should be savoring the fresh novelty of the morning.

I realized a few years ago that no matter what was going on in my life, unless I trained myself, I'd wake up thinking about what was *not* working in my life. It was a wake-up call. I decided I must develop a discipline to wake up thinking about what's working in my life and not what needs to be fixed. I tried many alternatives until I found one that increases my early-morning time in the focused mode.

Here is my first thought in the morning; it may help you, too.

☺   As soon as I wake up and become aware of myself and the world around me, I focus on gratitude. I start with a few deep breaths and think about five people in my life I'm grateful for. As I breathe in slowly and deeply, I bring the first person's face in front of my closed eyes. I try to see this person as clearly as I can in the part of the world where he or she is right now. Then I send this person my silent gratitude while breathing out — again, slowly and deeply. I repeat this exercise with five people. I avoid rushing through the experience, relishing the few seconds I spend remembering each person.

Waking up with gratitude helps me wake up to what's most important in my life. It gives context to my day. I wake up as a loving husband, father, son, brother, friend, colleague or neighbor, rather than someone running away from or toward deadlines, or feeling overwhelmed by life's challenges, both real and imaginary. I wake up feeling loved rather than feeling insecure.

I have a few additional suggestions to help keep your attention in the focused mode early in the morning. Please edit the specifics to match your experience.

☺   After completing the gratitude exercise, bring attention to your body and, feeling its stiffness, give it a stretch. If you share the bed with someone, look at that person, or if he or she is already out of bed, look where that person was sleeping with kind, soft eyes.

When you step out of bed, as your feet land on the floor, feel the floor's texture. Rub your feet against it, as if you are feeling it after a long time. As you walk toward the bathroom, continue feeling the floor against your feet and reconnect with the room.

In the bathroom, pay attention to the fragrance of potpourri. Look at your reflection with kindness and acceptance. Attend to at least one item decorating your sink pedestal. Maybe there's a silk plant you haven't seen for a month or a liquid soap bottle that has a lovely design worth paying attention to. As you brush your teeth, enjoy the flavor of the toothpaste.

In the shower, focus on the warm water touching your skin. Hum your favorite tune if you feel up to it. Pick up the soap and smell its rich fragrance. Pause for a few seconds and let the world stop as you feel the water falling on your head, trickling off your body. Imagine grace flowing into your home with the stream of water. Mentally visualize the river or creek from where this water came. As you dab yourself, feel the towel's dry surface on your skin.

Do not expect perfection in this exercise. Ruminations while you brush your teeth or shower are common and sometimes even creative. To begin with, if your only change is to practice gratitude first thing in the morning, that will suffice.

I find this exercise practical and helpful for many reasons. On the next page, read through the reasons listed and check yes if you agree with the questions that follow.

1. The exercise starts my day on a positive note. Would you like to start your day on a positive note? ❏ Yes   ❏ No
2. Gratitude connects me with the people I care most about. Would you like to connect with the people you care most about first thing in the morning? ❏ Yes   ❏ No
3. I feel nurtured when I think of people who care about me. Would you like to feel nurtured first thing in the morning? ❏ Yes   ❏ No
4. The exercise trains my attention so that I choose what I focus on. Would you like to train your attention so that you can choose what to focus on? ❏ Yes   ❏ No
5. Gratitude provides perspective on what's most important in my life. Would you like to think about what's most important in your life? ❏ Yes   ❏ No
6. I avoid visiting too many black holes and open files. Would you like to avoid visiting black holes and open files early in the morning? ❏ Yes   ❏ No
7. The exercise costs me minimal time. Would you like to get all of these benefits with a minimal time commitment? ❏ Yes   ❏ No

Can you think of any other benefits of such an exercise? Note them below.

Note: If you prefer, you can do this exercise with other gifts in your life, such as health, clean air, home, food, water or a safe neighborhood, instead of people. Personally, I find thinking about people as the most powerful draw to my attention.

Are there any good reasons you shouldn't practice this or a similar exercise? Try to counter those reasons with your good judgment.

Reason not to do the exercise	Counterargument

One common problem is forgetting. Most people want to practice gratitude but can't remember to do it. If this happens to you, here's a suggestion.

☺ Make a collage of pictures of the most important people in your life and post it on your bedroom wall so that you see it first thing in the morning. It will cue you to start your day with gratitude. If creating a collage takes too much effort, write the word *gratitude* on two sticky notes and post one on the bedroom wall and the other on the bathroom mirror. If you see the bathroom note before thinking about gratitude, go back to bed and start over.

Inserting a cue will do wonders to help you develop a new habit. After years of practice, I am addicted to the morning gratitude exercise, more than tea or coffee. I invite you to become an addict, too — a gratitude addict!

Exercise 2: Rx — Nature Once a Day (and as Needed)

Do you have access to nature or a natural environment close to your home or work?

Yes ❑   No ❑

When was the last time you spent some time in nature, remaining fully attentive to it? Or more specifically, how often do you spend time in nature, remaining fully attentive?

❑ Every day
❑ A few times a week
❑ A few times a month
❑ Rarely

Most people I meet have access to nature but don't pay attention to it. I am guilty as charged!

Before making any suggestions, I'll share the results of a few research studies:

▶ Walking in nature was associated with remarkable improvement in self-esteem and symptoms of depression compared with spending time in a mall.
▶ Families had the lowest stress when they were together in the backyard.
▶ Patients recovering from gallbladder surgery who had a view of trees from their hospital beds had shorter hospital stays and needed less pain medication compared with patients looking at a brick wall.
▶ Patients with burns who were shown a video program of scenic beauty combined with music experienced lower pain and anxiety when their dressings were changed compared with patients not shown such a program.

- Sunlight exposure is linked to lower stress.
- In patients with heart disease, exposure to nature was associated with a shorter length of stay and improved survival.

These results are partly because of a useful instinct: When we are in natural surroundings without a threat, we become relaxed and happy. Scientists call this the *positivity offset*. This instinct helps us explore, engage and interact. Hiking gives you a high, partly because of the positivity offset. With so many good reasons, why not spend at least some time every week admiring the trees and watching squirrels and bunnies in the yard? Spend a few minutes each day attending to nature. Start with this exercise.

☺   Look at the green grass, the blue sky, and the sizes and shapes of the clouds. Savor the color, the variety of plants and the squiggly tracks in the grass. Look at the plants and trees as selfless sages standing quietly, an emblem of peace, purifying air, holding the soil together, and giving us lovely flowers and fruits while asking nothing in return. Send them your silent gratitude for adorning your environment.

   Look at the tree's physical form — its height, branching pattern and the moss on the bark. Appreciate the shape and size of the green leaves and the pattern of the veins coursing through the leaves. Look at the bouquet of flowers and the squirrels and the birds finding shelter on the branches. Pay attention to the individual flowers. Attend to the color, shape and size of the petals. Notice how the petals are arranged in relation to each other. Appreciate the serrated (or smooth) edges of the leaves that surround the flower.

Nature tirelessly meets your every need, doesn't try to sell you a product, seeks nothing in return, and never negatively judges you by the way you dress or look. You can be yourself in nature — even on a bad hair day.

Compared with the before-screen era, we spend very little time in nature these days. With the growth of cities and screen time occupying a third of our day, nature has fallen to the back burner. I invite you to treat yourself to at least 10 to 15 minutes every day with nature.

Nature includes everything that's part of life and living systems or supports them — plants, trees, animals, oceans, rivers, lakes, creeks, hills, valleys, clouds, sky. A weed poking through the pavement also qualifies. Each of these provides a 3-D multisensory experience. On a day when the temperature is 30 degrees below zero, you can include indoor artwork or even music in your definition of nature.

Remember this instruction: When in nature, try not to plan or solve problems. Pay full attention to the external world. One way to do this is to pick a single flower, tree, leaf or even a blade of grass and try to fully know it. I have provided an exercise to do this in *The Mayo Clinic Guide to Stress-Free Living* on page 52.

Before you read further, mark your calendar when, later today or tomorrow, you'll spend some time in nature alone or preferably with people you care about.

Exercise 3: Heartfully Meet Loved Ones and Friends
Consider these two contrasting scenarios at the end of a workday.

Story 1: Mom arrives home around 5:30 p.m. from work, balancing grocery bags and a mountain of mail. She greets her 12-year-old, but he hardly notices, lost in an online game with his buddy from Malta, who he has never met or talked to. Her 17-year-old daughter has her back toward the room and is busy texting, watching a video online, downloading songs from the Internet, doing home-work and drinking an energy drink to help her focus. Dad arrives 20 minutes later. Mom and Dad share a hello; Dad and kids barely notice each other. The Red Sox are playing the Yankees today; Dad sits, excited, in front of the TV with a bag of popcorn, a bag of chips and a box of pretzels. In the next 10 minutes, he downs 1,200 calories. Dad skips dinner, Mom eats on the fly, and the kids eat while updating their social media accounts. By 8 p.m., Mom is exhausted and ready to go to bed. Dad is animated — the Sox won 5 to 4. He takes a sleeping pill to calm down. The kids finish their homework while chatting on the phone. The evening comes to a close.

Story 2: As soon as Mom comes home from work, the kids stop what they're doing and welcome her with a hug. Mom and kids share a snack and pick up a casual conversation. All eyes brighten as they hear the garage door open: Dad is home! They open the mudroom door to welcome him. The family sits down for a few minutes to swap stories. Dad pushes the red button on the digital video recorder to record the baseball game. Together, everyone walks into the kitchen. Dad starts cutting ingredients for the salad, Mom warms up the soup and stir-fries vegetables, and the kids set the table. The family spends the next 45 minutes enjoying a "happy meal," cracking jokes, chatting about sweet nothings, and sharing the best and the worst parts of their days. At the end of the dinner, the kids clean up the table and Dad loads the dishwasher. It's 7 p.m. Mom still has time to do the laundry while Dad checks the mail and returns some phone calls. They watch TV together. She falls asleep halfway through the game. Dad covers her legs with a blanket and shares a good-night hug with the kids. The evening comes to a close.

Which experience is likely to be more nurturing?

❏ The distracted first
❏ The heartful second

How often are you able to choose at least a few elements of the second (heartful) option with your friends or family?

❏ Every day
❏ A few times a week
❏ A few times a month
❏ Rarely

If you answered "rarely" or "a few times a month," you are in the majority. Of the tens of thousands of people I have polled, less than 5 percent consistently live the second (heartful) option. Most people I talk to experience work-related mind-wanderings for several hours after they get home.

Let's list the reasons people don't choose the heartful (and happier) option more often. Check each one that applies for you.

❏ Don't care about it
❏ Too busy
❏ Takes too much effort
❏ Stuck in open files at the end of the day
❏ Busy with the gadgets
❏ Live alone
❏ Don't get along with family
❏ Not in the habit
❏ Never thought about it
❏ Other _____
❏ Other _____
❏ Other _____

These are all good reasons to take a detour from living a fulfilled life. An average family reunites for only about 90 seconds at the end of the day before everyone gets busy in individual activities. And even when people choose to spend time together, their brains are still unavailable, busy with all of their open files. Now, let me share the five key ingredients that, when added to the mix, can make the heartful option a reality.

1. Wake up to novelty. Imagine sitting in a coffee shop with your spouse or partner. Your high school buddy walks up to your table. Who will you find more interesting for the next five minutes?

❏ Your spouse or partner
❏ Your high school buddy

I'm sure you said your high school buddy. Why is that? It's because of the perception of novelty. After years of togetherness, your loved ones often become familiar — even uninteresting — while your high school buddy immediately draws your attention. When pitched against love, novelty almost always will win your attention. Even in a loving relationship, perceived lack of novelty dries up the joy. Do you think that finding your loved ones novel will deepen your love?

Now think about being away on a 30-day trip alone. You don't get a chance to see your loved ones for that time. When you come back home, are you more likely to meet your clan with a more heartful presence, at least for the first 15 to 20 minutes?

Yes ❏   No ❏

Most people say yes to this question. Assuming you agree, what's different after 30 days? Check all that apply.

❏ I missed them.
❏ I'm excited to see them again.
❏ I find them new and interesting.
❏ I'm less likely to argue after several days of separation.
❏ There's more stuff to share.
❏ I've forgotten why I was angry with them.
❏ Other _____
❏ Other _____
❏ Other _____

Recognize what happens in the background. When you see your loved ones every day, they become familiar, almost boring. When you see them after 30 days, your system perceives one attribute that draws every mind's attention: novelty. The separation infuses fresh newness. Nothing changes, but the mutual perception of novelty is dialed up after the separation.

With this said, here's a question for you. If your loved ones are novel after you've been away for 30 days, are they novel each morning and evening? The answer is yes. Every day, everyone around you is fresh like morning dew. The novelty you see after 30 days of separation is simply the cumulative novelty built up each day. Based on what you've learned, here is your challenge and exercise.

☺   Can you meet your loved ones at the end of each day as if you're meeting them after 30 days? As you enter your home, tell yourself, *I am now going to meet a few very special people I haven't met for quite some time.* It's a new beginning, renewed connection, a fresh relationship being developed. You're more aware in their precious presence. You're kind; it's a moment of celebration. Can you challenge yourself to do a microcelebration when you meet your loved ones at the end of the day? I invite you to try this today.

To me, this is meditation.

> ✍ **Food for Thought:** Every day, everyone around you is fresh
> like morning dew. ☙

2. Try not to change others (acceptance). Here's your challenge for the next week: When you come home at the end of the day, try not to improve anybody for the first 3 minutes. Accept the living-room clutter, unfinished homework, unsorted mail, unpaid bills and even hair that's been dyed pink for the first 3 minutes. Why do I ask you to take this challenge? Picture yourself in this next situation and think about how you'd feel.

You are a homemaker with three busy children, ages 8, 7 and 4. After your spouse leaves for work at 7 a.m., you wake up the kids, get them ready for school and child care, pack their lunches and drop them off. You do the laundry, pay some bills, return a few phone calls, buy groceries and practice yoga for 30 minutes. It's already late afternoon. You drive back to pick up your kids, serve them a healthy snack, give the younger one a bath, take them for activities, prepare dinner and barely find some time to take a shower. It's now 7 p.m. Your kids are running around. The living room is a mess. Right then, your spouse comes home from work. With raised eyebrows, your spouse reacts by asking, "What have you done all day?"

In the box below, write how you would feel. Please avoid curse words!

We come with powerful fault-finding software installed within us. Your spouse used that software right away and forgot the important wisdom: You stop enjoying what you are trying to improve. It's a perfect way to distance ourselves from our loved ones.

Take this example and fast-forward six months. The spouse takes a course to improve relationships and puts it into practice. Now, the moment he gets home, he joins the kids in play. He creates a game around straightening up the living room. He helps you fix dinner. He appreciates how busy you are and coaches the kids to create less chaos.

Which response will help you enjoy clearing the chaos the next day, before he comes home?

❑ The first, judgmental response
❑ The second, nonjudgmental response

The skill he learned is to delay judgment by inviting greater acceptance. He has given up the urge to make others better. He has realized that nonacceptance pushes others away from him. His judgmental response makes both him and others unhappy. He knows that with nonacceptance, his loved ones associate his presence with feeling bad about themselves. His children may think, *I was feeling pretty good about myself until Dad showed up on the scene. Next time he comes home, I will make myself busy.* With this thinking, your loved ones won't blossom in your presence. That's a high price to pay.

Countless times I have heard my patients tell me that their best childhood memories are of their grandparents lighting up with joy when they saw them. Take this as a cue and light up when you see your family and friends. Delay the urge to improve others the moment you see them. Wouldn't it be nice to give the gift of acceptance to your loved ones? The best way to change others is to try not to change them. Accept them as they are. Your acceptance will provide them the incentive to become better than they are.

> 🕊 **Food for Thought:** The best way to change others is to try not to change them. 🕊

3. Appreciate transience. Let's assume you see your 70-year-old mother four times a year. How many more times will you see her in this life? If she lives to age 85, about 60 more times. That's all! I invite you to do this math with the people who are closest to you.

Person	Current age	Years we will be together*	Times we meet each year	Times we will meet in this life
Example: Mother	70	15	4	60

* Subtract the current age from 85. Use another number in place of 85 if it's more appropriate for your situation.

Our shared moments are finite — fewer than we think. Being aware of this finiteness brings greater meaning into our lives. You become kinder and less judgmental, which gives you permission to step out of daily chores and experience the joy of togetherness. You become more generous in giving your most precious gift: undivided attention.

We remain oblivious to transience. We pick squabbles for minor frustrations, living as if we have a blank check of infinite togetherness. The time to engage with your life is now. Tomorrow, your baby won't need your shoulder for comfort, your sixth-grader will know how to handle her homework and your teenager will have recovered her self-esteem.

Life isn't about success; it's about finding meaning in the obstructions to success. Seize your memorable moments before they depart unappreciated while you were busy checking emails. Make each moment count. Remembering transience almost always brings me into intentional presence.

> ✎ **Food for Thought:** Seize your memorable moments before they
> depart unappreciated while you were busy checking emails.
> Make each moment count. ✎

Keeping transience in mind, make note of some ways to enhance the quality of your time with the people you care most about below and on the next page.

Person	Relationship to me	Things I will do more often	Things I will do less often

Person	Relationship to me	Things I will do more often	Things I will do less often

The purpose of realizing transience isn't to stew over this thought and get depressed. It is to think about transience once in a while and use this awareness to find other people more meaningful.

4. Be flexible. In the evening, you crave quiet time with an interesting book and a cup of tea. But your 10-year-old wants to play ball, and your younger child has to be held. Your spouse reminds you of the leaky faucet in the basement, and moments later, a telemarketer tests your patience. What will you do?

❑ Shut everyone out and spend my hour with my book and a cup of tea.
❑ Do what has to be done, but with resignation, wishing to be left alone.
❑ Choose to engage with what is, balancing my need with the needs of others.

Isn't the third option the most practical and the one most conducive to long-term peace? Shutting everyone out may work for a day or two, but eventually it will backfire. Accommodating others' needs and preferences with resignation will fill your life with boredom and mediocrity. Choosing to engage with what is with cheerfulness will make you flexible.

By being flexible, you avoid disharmony and ego battles. Be flexible about the choice of soup for dinner, on which side of the bed you sleep, and most certainly with the color of the hair clip your daughter should wear. Talk to your teenagers about what interests them instead of what interests you. Slowly, they will start associating you with feeling good about themselves and will open up. All of the minor preferences aren't worth fighting over. Remember how much you wanted to press the elevator button when you were a child. Look at others' minor preferences as the elevator buttons that are still important to them. This will help you be flexible. Your flexibility is the perfect gift that will sustain joy in your family.

5. Say one good thing. Authentic praise is based on two key understandings:

- I like people who like me.
- I like myself when I like people.

Most of us depend on the appreciation of others to feel good about ourselves. How you view yourself is the sum total of how you think others see you. Which of the following sentences sounds like music to your ears?

- ❑ Sandra, you were right when you said . . .
- ❑ Bob, I can't thank you enough for your advice on . . .
- ❑ Josh, you are such a good father to . . .
- ❑ Mom, I can never forget how lovingly you helped me when . . .

You probably liked all of them. We all feel good when we are reminded of our goodness.

Our first experience of love is unconditional. As a baby, you receive authentic love that has no expectations. Try to give that love to others by saying something good about them.

Make an effort to find what's right in others. When you search for goodness, you'll invariably find it. It'll help you admire people. Your admiration will inspire them to find what's right in you, creating a nurturing exchange that may last a lifetime. The best way to impress is to be impressed.

With children, focus on respect in addition to love. Seldom do children hear that they are respected. Your respect for children's good behavior will inspire them to make it a habit. Children also crave validation, particularly from adults. Research shows that the one solid anchor that makes children resilient is attention from an adult who believes in them, shows love and respect, and is trustworthy. That adult doesn't always have to be a parent. It could be a neighbor, teacher, friend's parent, priest or even a grocer. This is particularly true for disadvantaged children. You could be a mentor for many precious lives.

☺ When you meet your loved ones today, let your job in the first five minutes be to find something nice about them and creatively say it. Be authentic rather than picking a cliché. Your authentic praise will make their day and yours, too.

One word of caution, though. Avoid sudden transformation. If overnight you suddenly dial up your warmth from room temperature to 350 degrees and start meeting your spouse or partner every day with long passionate hugs, kisses and unreal excitement, your partner might find it weird. The purpose isn't to shock and awe. The idea is to intelligently engage a part of your loved one's brain that he or she enjoys visiting. Show that you are in a good mood. If you are crabby, others (particularly children) think they've done something wrong. In your presence, they'll spin a cocoon and close themselves in. The cocoon hardens with time, but rest assured, even the hardest cocoons have soft areas. Find your loved ones novel and help them find you novel. Appreciate and be honest and creative about your appreciation, which you will be if you're authentic.

Intelligent admiration speaks volumes. It says that you're happy, present, attentive and appreciative—all very beneficial to a loving, nurturing relationship. Each person has a child within waiting to be tickled awake. Help others feel the innocence and joy of being a child. Think of the fondest memories of your childhood. Are they related to getting the most expensive toy? Or do they remind you of the times you felt loved and accepted? If it's the latter, wouldn't it be nice to create many more of these moments for yourself and others? Your resolve to give these moments is the first and most essential step on this journey.

If you're single. You don't have to be married or have a loving partner to practice these ideas. You can give similar attention to your friends, neighbors, clients, customers and even pets. Pets — dogs, in particular — see you as novel each time you meet them. So do 2-year-olds. Only an hour of separation is enough for them to press the refresh button. This is a basic instinct that we lose as we grow up. I think it's a great loss.

At work. I suggest developing a two-step process when meeting someone in a work setting. First, meet the person simply as a person. Do not immediately see others as a means to an end; try to first know them as fellow human beings, if only for 30 seconds. Then meet the person as your client. Spending even a few seconds seeing someone simply as a person will make meeting your client more rewarding and enjoyable.

Seeing novelty in others will connect you with the world at a deeper level. It'll help you experience greater joy. If this isn't meditation, then I don't know what is.

Additional Ideas for Practice

Several additional practices are beneficial for training attention. The goal with any of these practices is to find extraordinary within ordinary. Practices for training attention are listed below and described in the appendix.

1. Find uniqueness within the ordinary.
2. Use one sensory system at a time.
3. Find one new detail (FOND).
4. Contemplate the story.

When you get a chance, read about these attention-training exercises and see if any of them interest you.

Next, we'll integrate these ideas into a structured program. My goal is to offer an approach that is simple, intuitive and practical for your life.

> 🕊 **Food for Thought:** Seeing novelty in others
> will connect you with the world at a deeper level.
> It'll help you experience greater joy. 🕊

Joyful Attention: A Structured Approach

Over the years, I've found that I need discipline and structure to tame my un-yielding mind. Maybe this is true for you, too. This structured approach can help you improve your joyful attention skills and invite greater happiness into your life. It progresses in two phases: train it and sustain it.

Phase 1: Train It

Your attention is like a muscle: Training makes it stronger. Since you may have to undo your mind's lifelong tendency to wander, greater discipline and rigor early on (without being nerdy) will help. The Train It phase lasts anywhere from four to 24 weeks, depending on your effort and natural attention skills. Since sustaining joyful attention throughout the day is impractical, I suggest sprinkling moments of focusing your attention throughout your day.

> Practice joyful attention three or four times a day during the Train It phase. The best times include when waking up in the morning, at breakfast, at the start of a meeting, while listening to a presentation, during lunch, while connecting with nature, when arriving home from work, at family time in the evening, at the dinner table, before you go to sleep, in church and at other times that fit your schedule.

Turn to the next page for a summary of three practices that invites you to make a promise to yourself to practice joyful attention.

Joyful attention practices	Sounds like a good idea	I can do it
Wake up with gratitude and in the moment	❏	❏
Start my day with five thoughts of gratitude	❏	❏
Feel the floor under my feet	❏	❏
Be aware of something interesting in the bathroom	❏	❏
Pause during my shower to enjoy water on my skin	❏	❏
Imagine grace flowing into my home with water	❏	❏
Attend to nature (the physical world)	❏	❏
Spend quality time in the backyard	❏	❏
Visit a playground	❏	❏
Walk in my neighborhood	❏	❏
Get to know a tree	❏	❏
Attend to a flower	❏	❏
Appreciate indoor artwork	❏	❏
Heartfully meet my loved ones and friends	❏	❏
Pay attention to what makes them unique	❏	❏
Appreciate transience	❏	❏
Try not to change others	❏	❏
Keep flexible preferences	❏	❏
Be cheerful when I meet my loved ones	❏	❏
Find reasons to praise them	❏	❏

Beyond these times of active practice, try to pay greater attention to the world around you throughout the day. Study the design of a book's cover, the shape of a doorknob, patterns on the countertop, cracks in the pavement, colors of the elevator buttons, sprinklers on the ceiling, peeling paint from the wall — all of these are worth paying attention to. Each time you intentionally attend to the ordinary, you engage and train your brain's focused mode.

After the initial four to 24 weeks, your active need for formal practice might wane as you increasingly anchor in an attention pattern that's flexible, relaxed and nonjudgmental. The formal exercises will give way to effortless practice throughout the day. What was initially a goal becomes the path, and eventually, a habit. You will then be in the Sustain It phase.

Phase 2: Sustain It

This phase lasts for the rest of your life as you sustain the gains you've realized by training your attention and find different ways to engage it. The rate of progress varies from person to person. Your goal is to advance from a transient state of calm to a transformed stage in which intentional attention to novelty and goodness in others is as natural to you as breathing. With practice, you'll meet many more people during the day with joyful attention, creating multiple micromoments of happiness. A few moments of practice will create a new habit. Gradually these moments will bridge together, lifting your entire day. You'll become more alive.

In this time, I invite you to choose a new activity, such as arts and crafts, a cooking class, yoga, Pilates or music. A novel activity will help you focus your attention, and in turn, the activity will benefit from your stronger focus.

As you achieve deeper attention, I suggest still taking time for a few elements of disciplined daily practice. Discipline will prevent you from reverting to your earlier state of mind-wandering and will deepen your experience. As you advance in your practice, you'll be much better attuned with your particular needs and will carve out a program that best fits with your life.

A program to deepen your attention will awaken the child within you. Part of the reason children have so much fun is because they can find novelty within the ordinary. They have a long list of things that are interesting to them. As we get older, that list shortens. Don't let that happen to you. By practicing joyful attention, your list can grow again, gifting you with more moments when you are joyous and fully alive.

After four weeks of practice, visit the checklist on page 70 and note which ideas you were able to apply and which you will continue.

Attention exercises	Able to practice	Will continue
Wake up with gratitude and in the moment	❑	❑
Attend to nature	❑	❑
Heartfully meet my loved ones and friends	❑	❑
(List additional practice.)	❑	❑
(List additional practice.)	❑	❑
(List additional practice.)	❑	❑

After learners complete initial attention training, I encourage them to start a daily 15-minute program of deep breathing, progressive muscular relaxation or guided imagery. I have provided a few sample exercises in Week 9. If you're interested in deeper (sitting) meditation, I suggest a more individualized approach with help from an experienced instructor.

If you like to track your progress using a journal, visit *www.stressfree.org*, go to the Resources tab and find journal pages that you can print and use.

Joyful Attention: A Few Words of Advice

Now, I'd like to share three suggestions I have found useful over the years for training attention.

1. Find Empty Time

Research shows that an average person has more than 150 undone tasks at any time. If you're an average person, you're very busy. I have a suggestion for finding time to practice training your attention.

Inventory your day and identify times that aren't very productive, when what you're doing needs only a fraction of your brain's capacity. These are the times when your attention is likely to drift. Remind yourself to convert these times to moments of joyful attention.

❏ Standing in an elevator
❏ Walking to the cafeteria
❏ Folding the laundry
❏ Doing the dishes
❏ Waiting for the computer to boot up
❏ Waiting on hold on the phone
❏ Standing in the grocery line
❏ Waiting for a meeting to start
❏ Waiting to pick up my child at school
❏ Warming up my breakfast
❏ Other _____
❏ Other _____

Recognize that joyful attention practices are designed so that they won't take extra time. They are integrated into your life. You aren't adding more milk to your already full cup; instead, you're adding chocolate powder to your milk. You wake up every day and spend time in the bathroom. Why not practice gratitude and train your brain in that time? You meet your loved ones and others at the end (or beginning) of the day. Why not bring a more authentic and complete presence in that time? By minimizing how much your mind wanders, and with practice, these simple exercises may *save* you time, instead of costing any.

2. Improve Your Overall Well-Being

It takes energy to train your attention. On the next page, you'll find ideas that'll help you be kind to your entire being as you progress along this path. Find additional ideas to unlock your energy in Week 10. Look through the list on the next page. Check the ones that resonate with you and make a plan to do them.

Activity	Sounds like a good idea	How I will do it
Adequate sleep	❏	
Healthy diet	❏	
Active body (exercise)	❏	
Improved relationships	❏	
Volunteer activity	❏	
Other	❏	
Other	❏	
Other	❏	

3. Involve Others

Find a buddy who can walk with you on this journey. Your buddy can be your spouse or partner, adult child, parent, co-worker, or anyone who is also interested in learning the skills of the Resilient Living Program. When working with someone, remember that you can only teach yourself. Others learn by seeing you learn. A common mistake is to start negatively judging others who aren't interested in pursuing these or other mind-body approaches. Such judgment will push you away from them and slow your progress. Teach less, embody more.

> 🦢 **Food for Thought:** Others learn by seeing you learn.
> Teach less, embody more. 🦢

While you may be excited about focusing on what makes other people unique, they may still be stuck in a lifelong pattern of distracted attention, screen addiction or both. This is a barrier that many people face. I have two suggestions if you find yourself in this situation.

☺   **Be creative.** Creatively plan your attention-training activities so that your loved ones associate you with novelty and feeling good about themselves. For starters, consider filling your evening with at least one activity that brings your family together — share a glass of wine with your significant other, play ball with the kids, jump rope together, bring home your family's favorite food, participate in small talk, watch a TV show together — any of these will do. Be flexible to accommodate others' preferences. While the specifics may be different for all of us and may change from one day to the next, any gesture that helps others feel appreciated and cared for, and their uniqueness accepted and admired, will work.

     Be patient. Patience is your gift to others. Hurry is almost always internal. A mind in a hurry races past the present. When you have to wait longer than you would like, fill that time with joyful attention by noticing the details of the world around you. It'll prevent you from being impatient.

Whatever you do, be kind — to yourself and others. That's where it all starts. One way to enhance your kindness is to practice kind attention, our next step.

TRY THIS TODAY

Make a collage of the most important people in your life and post the collage on your bedroom wall so that you see it first thing in the morning. It will cue you to start your day with gratitude. If creating a collage takes too much effort, write the word *gratitude* on two sticky notes and post one on the bedroom wall and another on the bathroom mirror. This cue will help you develop your gratitude habit.

Week 2: Kind Attention

Imagine this scenario. It's past midnight. Your car is parked on a dark street corner and has a flat tire. While mentally going over the steps for changing the tire, you see two 6-foot-5-inch, 300-pound shadows lumbering toward you. How do you respond?

- ❏ I start munching on potato chips.
- ❏ I step out and hug the two men.
- ❏ I turn on my favorite music.
- ❏ I call 911.

I would call 911 ASAP. A word about the human brain's fear center will help put this experience into perspective. The information coming into your brain is screened for threat by its almond-sized fear center called the amygdala. Snakes, spiders, tigers, armed strangers — all these activate our amygdalae to alert us to danger. This instinct helped us survive the million different challenges that our ancestors faced.

Instincts die hard. Research in the modern world shows that our amygdalae scan people's faces. Anyone threatening or different fires up the amygdala. Individual responses vary; some of us are more afraid of strangers than others are.

A milder version of this instinct makes us launch snap judgments about others the moment we see them. Take a 10-minute stroll in the mall. Five people will have created a story about you in their heads. Research shows that in a 10th of a second, we make conclusions about other people's trustworthiness, competence, aggressiveness, attractiveness and likability. And although many of these judgments are wrong, we remain confident about our quick conclusions. Since we now live in communities that range from a few thousand to millions of people as opposed to a few hundred in a tribe, the countless judgments we have to make each day as a result can leave our brains busy and feeling fatigued.

We must soften this instinct of rapid-fire judgments if we wish to be peaceful. Kind attention is a step toward that.

Instinctive Attention

You can see others with three different sets of eyes. The first two are instinctive, and the third can be trained in kind attention. Untrained attention commonly sees others with:

1. Neutral eyes, with little attention (busy with a wandering mind).
2. Judgmental eyes that—
    ▶ Size people up by focusing on physical attributes such as clothes, body structure or attractiveness (particularly with the opposite sex)
    ▶ Assess possible threats

When you judgmentally focus on the physical details or perceived threat, you deplete yourself of vital energy. I believe every time you see another person, you have an opportunity to feel good about yourself using a third set of eyes. Learn how, starting on the next page.

Kind Attention

☺ When you see someone, don't allow your mind to make judgments. Instead, recognize that each person is dealing with his or her own struggles. Align your heart and eyes and send that person this silent blessing: *I wish you well.*

You can consider it a two-second prayer. By understanding how the human brain and mind work, you *know* that every person has numerous unresolved concerns and uncertainties. You recognize what Henry Wadsworth Longfellow said: "If we could read the secret history of our enemies, we should find in each man's life sorrow and suffering enough to disarm all hostility."

Kind attention is thus a two-way process. You send positive energy into the world as you take in information.

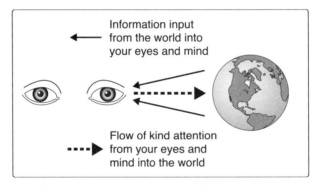

Information input from the world into your eyes and mind

Flow of kind attention from your eyes and mind into the world

Kind attention: A two-way flow of energy

Kind attention looks at everyone with the third set of eyes: kind eyes. Three different beliefs help me look at the world with kind eyes. Below and on the next page, choose the option that resonates best with you.

Understanding	Kind eyes	Personal favorite
Everyone struggles with unresolved issues.	Send a silent blessing: *I wish you well.*	❏

Understanding	Kind eyes	Personal favorite
Each person means a lot to someone; everyone has a network of people that cares for him or her.	See the other person from within his or her circle of love. Imagine you are part of that circle.	❏
Every human has the same spiritual essence as you.	See others as equal to you in their spiritual essence and potential.	❏

Kind Attention: FAQs

People often ask me the following four questions about kind attention.

Do I need to say something in order to give kind attention?

The practice is designed to be silent. You wish others well in the privacy of your mind. You can reserve saying, "Bless you" for the times when people sneeze.

I am shy and introverted and don't like to look strangers in the eye. Is eye contact necessary for kind attention?

Eye contact isn't necessary. You can see someone coming from the other direction and send kind attention without knowing who that person is or how he or she looks.

How can I send kind attention in an unsafe neighborhood when I myself am afraid?

You don't have to. Start with a familiar place, where you feel safe, and with people you care about. As you grow, your circle of kind attention will expand.

What are the benefits of kind attention?

There are several. You wish yourself well when you wish others well. Your kind attention reflects as soft eyes, a smile on your face and a gentle voice. People recognize your kindness even when they don't see you, such as when you're talking on the phone. The only person hurt by your judgmental eyes is you. When you look at others with kind eyes, the practice creates a feeling of love in you. It gives you multiple opportunities to experience positive emotions during the day. It also trains your brain to be in the focused mode and helps you delay judgment. You like yourself when you like others.

🖎 **Food for Thought:** You like yourself when you like others. 🖎

You have a choice: don't pay attention, allow judgmental attention or choose kind attention. Ask yourself: How would you like others to look at you? Do you want them to judge you or accept you as you are? If it's the latter, practice kind attention for the next few days and come back to this page and write about how it felt.

I have tried kind attention for _____ days.
Describe your experience.

I dream of living in a world that looks at my children with kind attention. I suppose that's true for you, too. Let's join hands and create such a society around us. It has to start somewhere. Why not with you and me?

🖎 **Food for Thought:** Look at the world as you want the world to look at your children and other loved ones. 🖎

TRY THIS TODAY

When you see someone, don't allow your mind to make judgments or focus on how he or she looks physically. Instead, align your heart and eyes and send that person this silent blessing: *I wish you well.*

The Second Step: Cultivate Emotional Resilience

Weeks 3–8: Flow with Life's Stressors

On any given day, the odds are good that you'll encounter stressors. Research shows that an average person experiences significant stressors three to four days a week.

Maybe you're late to work, you receive an angry email or your daughter's child care provider is ill and you have to make other arrangements at the last minute. You want to be emotionally resilient so that you can negotiate these challenging situations with relative ease. You want to withstand and bounce back from adversity as fast as you can.

Weeks 3–8 of this program are designed to give you tools and strategies you can use at any given time to refocus your thoughts away from your feelings of stress and toward productive ways of working with life's stressors. These approaches will enhance your inner strength by making you emotionally resilient and happier.

Emotional resilience means:

- Experiencing positive emotions on most days
- Preserving emotional stability through adversity
- Recovering positive emotions quickly after facing adversity

Emotionally resilient people engage in and savor life's experiences without overindulging. They exercise appropriate caution without excessive fear. They have a healthy sense of self without being arrogant. They don't seek perfection, aren't in denial, and aren't overly optimistic or pessimistic. They embrace their vulnerabilities, work with what is and are flexible about their preferences.

We'll start Weeks 3 through 8 by talking about the key ingredients of emotional resilience. This will lead to five principles to practice and use in your daily life that will help you not only enhance your emotional resilience but also improve your focus and creativity and deepen your engagement with life — and teach you skills that you can apply to most life situations.

Emotional Resilience: The Ingredients

My mother keeps a special curry powder at home. It's a mix of curry leaves, sun-dried mangoes, ginger, chili, coriander, garlic, cloves, cardamom, cumin, fennel, sea salt, turmeric and mustard seeds. If any vegetable, soup or lentil preparation doesn't taste right, a few spoonfuls of this powder added to the mix always does the trick.

Several years ago, I started a project to make a different kind of curry powder — for the mind. I searched for a combination of principles that can soothe and possibly even transform most of life's stressors. After years of studying and experimenting, I found the perfect flavor with a mix of five ingredients:

1. Gratitude
2. Compassion
3. Acceptance
4. Meaning
5. Forgiveness

Together, these timeless principles provide the foundation for emotional resilience. You can learn about the background of these principles in *The Mayo Clinic Guide to Stress-Free Living.* Understanding the inner workings of your brain and mind, training your attention, and living according to higher principles are all ways to develop your emotional resilience. At the same time, these principles, when fully internalized, can also at least partially heal almost any emotional hurt. I invite you to bring them to your life.

First Steps

Let's play a game to introduce you to the principles. Imagine you're a teenager who really cares about how your hair looks. Your hairstylist completely messed up your haircut today. You are mad and want to shout your lungs out, but in five minutes, your boyfriend or girlfriend will pick you up for a date. That's all the time you have to cheer yourself up. In the following table, see five perspectives that might help. Try to match them with the principles in the right column.

1. Hairstylists have a tough job. They are expected to be right 100 percent of the time. After all, they're only human.	A. Gratitude B. Compassion C. Acceptance D. Meaning E. Forgiveness
2. Of the hundreds of haircuts I get, it shouldn't be a big deal if one goes bad. Few things in life go right more than 99 percent of the time.	
3. If my boyfriend or girlfriend still likes me with this crappy haircut, then he or she really cares about me for who I am.	
4. I have messed up so many projects myself. I remember spilling mayonnaise on a guest when I waited on a table. I should let this go and move on.	
5. I'm so lucky I have a scalp full of hair. It'll grow back in no time.	
Answers: 1. B 2. C 3. D 4. E 5. A	

Do you see how each principle and its related perspective can help you recover more quickly and is a different — and kinder — way of looking at the same thing? Do you see how the principles reframe the experience in its full context and can take you toward peace and happiness?

Applying these principles doesn't mean you deny the reality or stop taking care of yourself. Unbridled optimism or positivity can be counterproductive. Did I say the hairstyle looked good? No, because that isn't the truth. Your mind would repel that idea. The principles also don't ask you to go back to the same hairstylist. They are a more pragmatic way of looking at life, a faster approach to peace and quicker healing to help prevent this experience from spoiling the rest of your day. They help stop your fight with yourself.

You can't remove all undesirable experiences from your life. But you can become intentional about how you handle them and, in the end, reclaim control over your mind. With practice, you'll be able to apply the principles in more difficult situations than getting a bad haircut. This will provide you with a path toward lasting happiness.

A structured approach, with a theme for each day, will help you do this. I sometimes call this the flavor of the day. Here is a suggested sequence to use.

Day of the week	Theme (flavor of the day)
Monday	Gratitude
Tuesday	Compassion
Wednesday	Acceptance
Thursday	Meaning
Friday	Forgiveness
Saturday	Celebration
Sunday	Reflection or prayer

A disciplined practice for the first six weeks trains the mind to learn to use these principles. Most participants in the Resilient Living Program continue with this sequence after six weeks, and many plan to keep it for the rest of their lives. Next I briefly describe each principle.

Monday's Theme: Gratitude

Start your day by sending silent gratitude to at least five people, as you learned to do in the exercise on joyful attention. Through the day, particularly when your attention is pulled toward something unpleasant or undesirable, try to reframe your thoughts with gratitude. Instead of thinking, *I hate being so busy,* consider telling yourself, *I'm grateful I'm able to help so many.* If, for instance, you're a health care provider, you could focus on being grateful to your patients for the trust and respect they give to you and your profession. If you're a businessperson, you could be grateful to your clients for their confidence in you and the gift of their business. As a stay-at-home parent, you could be grateful for the comfort of your home and the priceless treasure of your children. Raising children with a balance of discipline and love is more important than any other job in the world. As a stay-at-home parent, you're employed in the hospitality industry and your customers happen to be your loved ones. What could be better than that?

When things go wrong, as they invariably will, try to focus on what went right within what went wrong. Consider being grateful that what happened wasn't as bad as what could have happened. It's often challenging to be grateful when you're buried under the rubble of adversity. But gratitude can open a much-needed crack to let the light in. With practice, your gratitude threshold changes. You become automatically grateful for the many little — and larger — gifts that life offers. Gratitude then cultivates an ever-present, cheerful calm in your mind. Gratitude stops being the goal. Instead, it adorns the entire path. Gratitude provides you with energy you can use to practice compassion.

🕊 **Food for Thought:** Try to focus on what went right
within what went wrong. 🕊

Tuesday's Theme: Compassion

Compassion is the practice of the golden rule. With compassion, you recognize that all of us struggle, are fighting little or large battles, and deserve each other's kindness. This is particularly true for the patients and their care providers, who feel vulnerable and experience lack of control, uncertainty and the rude realization of finiteness.

Compassion helps you remember that an expression other than love is a call for help. Someone may act ornery because she's hurt, though she may not say so. The simple formula is this:

upset = hurt = call for help

Food for Thought: An expression other than love is a call for help.

The alternative formula — upset = insult = call for reaction — perpetuates an unhealthy reaction that can damage your relationships.

With compassion, you truly see the other person from within his or her perspective. Annoyance is a symptom of unhappiness, unhappiness originates in hurts, and hurts sprout from an unmet expectation. Your counteranger will only further scrape his or her wounds. It'll increase annoyance, unhappiness and hurt and fuel further disappointment.

Compassion provides the healing balm to soothe the symptom and cure the disease. Compassion is the miracle lotion that can nurse the nastiest emotional sores back to health. Seeking compassion will make you happier than seeking happiness. Your compassion recognizes suffering, empathizes with it and cultivates an intention to relieve suffering. It leads you to take action to comfort and heal. Compassion isn't passive observation; it's a call for action, with passion.

Wednesday's Theme: Acceptance
Acceptance has three components:

1. Acceptance of others
2. Acceptance of yourself
3. Acceptance of situations

We can accept others (and ourselves) once we realize that all of us as humans have elements of imperfection and are fallible. We seek timeless wisdom and perfect love but are works in progress. We don't have a foolproof instruction manual for living. We learn by what life teaches us. Our thoughts and actions, although well meaning and altruistic, may still represent imbalanced fear, desire and ego. Acceptance of others originates in embracing these imperfections. You expand your worldview, ultimately recognizing that by accepting others, you accept yourself.

Being able to accept situations springs from the realization that the collective energy of the universe has many mouths to feed, and sometimes the clouds choose to rain elsewhere. Half of the earth has to face away from the sun for the other half to be bathed in sunlight. That's just the way it is. Acceptance allows you to preserve your hope and optimism so that you can truly believe that a step back is a move forward. This belief helps you engage with what's most meaningful rather than escape into the psychological time that's commonly filled with fatiguing what ifs.

Acceptance fosters inner calmness that'll stop you from fighting your own self and, as a result, save energy so that you have it when you need to respond to an external challenge. Acceptance helps you make happiness a priority even when you face adversity and disappointment. Acceptance helps you be fair and rational even on a day that may have invited chaos. It helps you be kind — predictably kind. Acceptance isn't apathy. It's empowered surrender, a state that balances passion and calmness with the wisdom of transience and justice.

Thursday's Theme: Meaning

In each moment, you do what's most meaningful to you at that moment. The three questions that help me summarize the meaning of my life are:

1. Who am I?
2. Why do I exist?
3. What is this world?

Who am I? I carry many identifiers. At work, I'm a professional, and at home or socially, I'm a husband, father, son, brother, colleague, neighbor and friend. Two threads join all of these roles and represent the true meaning of my life: *service* and *love*. No matter what I do or where I am, I can be of service and love. The same holds true for you. Service and love are complete in themselves. They'll be with you forever. While your roles may continue to evolve, no one can take away your right to be of service and love.

Why am I here? I exist to make this world a little kinder and happier than I found it. However small my contribution, I believe if we all keep this simple goal, many or most of our self-created problems will fade away. Each of us is given a small canvas of Mother Nature to decorate. Our job is to paint and bejewel it as best we can so that the next generation finds value and inspiration in it.

What is this world? This world is a school of learning. My life's blessings, both successes and failures, are lessons. They give me precious insight into the nature of reality. Thinking in this way helps me remain humble and flow with the hardships without personalizing my adversities or negative feedback.

Understanding the different aspects of meaning helps you focus more on the energy that you send to others than on the energy coming your way. Thursday is a day of low expectations filled with humility. It is a day to be pleasantly surprised and excited about each gift, small or large, coming your way. It's a day to make someone's life a little happier than it may have been otherwise. It is also the day when you realize that the ultimate meaning is experienced not in the confines of the past and the future, but in this very day, in the splendor of now.

Friday's Theme: Forgiveness

Most of us are at one of two poles in terms of forgiveness. At one end, forgiveness seems unnecessary because life has been blessed in so many ways. At the other end is unfairness, when someone has been hurt deeply. Both of these perceptions, for different reasons, push us away from the virtue of forgiveness.

Forgiveness is your willful choice to live life based on your highest ideals. It's your gift to others and ultimately to yourself. Forgiveness is essential for overcoming the spiritual stress tests that life sends your way. Forgiveness that is willful and mature is empowering and doesn't take away your strength or self-respect. Forgiveness frees up your mind to discover greater meaning and happiness.

Forgiveness is the end result of a concerted practice of gratitude, compassion, acceptance and pursuit of life's higher meaning. We forgive when we compassionately understand the human condition and when we realize that human minds are intrinsically driven by selfish cravings and dislikes. We forgive when we accept the good and bad in all of us, knowing that they're contextual and ever changing — what is bad today may seem good tomorrow.

We forgive because we want life's higher meaning — and not our hurts — to guide our journey.

Our forgiveness of others depends on forgiveness of ourselves. Forgiving yourself energizes your forgiveness of others, and vice versa. As we grow, make progress and begin to forgive the past, we also can start forgiving the future. In this journey, a time comes when the need to forgive dissolves. In that instant, we discover who we are, realizing that gratitude, compassion, acceptance, life's higher meaning and forgiveness are different names of the same force: love.

Themes for Saturday and Sunday: Celebration, Reflection or Prayer

Celebration and prayer are related to your individual lifestyle and beliefs, so I'll defer the specifics to your good judgment. Suffice it to say that flexible preferences, an inclusive outlook and a general flavor of unselfishness will enhance peace, joy and resilience, through work as well as play.

• • •

Can I practice all of these principles perfectly? Certainly not. But do I think I am better at it today than I was a decade ago? Absolutely. Progress is often slower than you wish, but it's progress nonetheless. And with this progress come the gifts of freedom — from hurtful negative emotions to greater happiness and better self-control. With practice, you have better influence over your mind and can choose your thoughts. That is a critical step in progress. When you choose your thoughts, they are healthier; when thinking happens to you, you are more likely to wander into negativity.

If you keep these themes through the day, you'll start doing ordinary things extraordinarily. Character is more determined by how you relate with the common and mundane and not particularly when the spotlight is on you.

You might ask, *Why not practice gratitude on Tuesday, too?* The purpose of a structured approach is to have a particular focus for each day, not to exclude other values. Please don't say on a Friday that you can't practice compassion today because that is limited to Tuesdays. In fact, with practice, you will realize that each of these values converges toward the same point. They are different flavors of the two core virtues from where all of this came: wisdom and love.

These suggested practices aren't meant to make you rigid. If you find a particular practice difficult, you can substitute it for another one that feels easier for you. Some learners focus on practicing gratitude all week. That's just fine. My goal is to provide a road map for happiness and resilience. The journey is yours to carve. But if you have no particular reason to choose otherwise, I suggest at least starting with this sequence: gratitude, compassion, acceptance, meaning, forgiveness, celebration, reflection or prayer.

Early in your practice, you might use these values as a way to reinterpret your negative experiences. These values are your quarterbacks when adversities launch an assault. As you advance, they may become the defining aspect of your day. The whole day may become one constant stream of gratitude, compassion, acceptance, higher meaning and forgiveness. How can suffering find home in such a being?

In the rest of this section, we will look at these principles in greater depth. We will look at each principle in three ways:

1. Understand the principle (what it is).
2. Find meaning in the principle (why you should practice it).
3. Apply the principle in your life (how to practice it).

> 🖋 **Food for Thought:** Character is determined more by how you relate with the common and mundane and not particularly when the spotlight is on you. 🖌

Through these steps, my ultimate goal is to help you make these principles your very own so that their practice becomes effortless. When you start inhaling gratitude and converting it to compassion and default to acceptance and forgiveness, you'll transform and lift the little universe that surrounds you.

The cognitive and emotional parts of your brain are like two wheels of a bike: They must work together. With synergy in your cognitive and emotional brains, you'll be able to apply the principles from the whole of your being. Let's start with gratitude.

Gratitude

Understanding Gratitude

Gratitude is acknowledging and appreciating your blessings. Gratitude is being blessed and knowing that you are blessed. Gratitude represents your thankfulness for every experience, because each step of life can help you grow — sometimes materially, but almost always emotionally and spiritually. Four conditions have to be met for you to feel grateful:

1. You receive something of value.
2. The giver shared it voluntarily, not out of obligation.
3. Sharing took effort on the part of the giver.
4. The giver shared it with no selfish intent.

Let's discuss the third and the fourth conditions.

The Giver Made an Effort to Share

How often have you felt deeply grateful that your grocery store stocks your favorite cereal? Let's call it the Yummy-Yum brand.

❏ Seldom, if ever
❏ Whenever I am buying it
❏ Whenever I am eating it
❏ Several times every day

Most people say "Seldom, if ever." Now consider this. Yummy-Yum cereal is in short supply. You settle for another brand. One afternoon, the grocery store manager leaves you a message. Knowing your preference, he has saved five boxes of your favorite cereal for you. You pick it up from the store. The cereal's price isn't marked up. Are you likely to feel grateful for the five boxes? Check yes or no.

Yes ❏   No ❏

If you answered yes, it's because of the extra attention and care you received. Special effort by someone on your behalf instills gratitude in you. If you answered no, it's either because you don't care so much about the cereal or because you are hard to please. I'm sure it's the former!

The Giver Shared It With No Selfish Intent
Consider this experience: You recently relocated to a new country and are feeling lonely. You run into an old acquaintance at the mall. He invites you for dinner the following weekend. When you show up, your acquaintance serves an elaborate multicourse meal. Will you feel grateful?

Yes ❑   No ❑

Halfway through the dinner, your acquaintance changes the topic to investments. He pressures you to buy into a financial scheme that you don't have the desire or resources to purchase. You politely decline, but he keeps pushing. Will your gratitude dampen at this point?

Yes ❑   No ❑

Finally, he relents, but now he is cold and distant. He chooses not to serve the dessert that you know was prepared. Write a few words about how you would feel in the space provided below.

```



```

I doubt you wrote many kind words. A selfish motive is the perfect annihilator of gratitude. At best, it makes you feel indebted.

Gratitude Versus Indebtedness

Whether you feel grateful or indebted depends on the intention. When you feel cared for, considered worthy and treated with kindness, with no expectations in return, you feel grateful. When help comes with a built-in expectation to repay, you feel indebted. Indebtedness feels heavy; it creates an obligation. Too much indebtedness feels as if you are carrying an extra mortgage. Gratitude is felt equally by the receiver and giver, while indebtedness only by the receiver. Gratitude is spiritual, while indebtedness is an ordinary business transaction.

Meaning in Gratitude

Imagine seeing your doctor for low energy and a depressed mood. After thorough evaluation, he prescribes a pill that research shows can boost your energy, improve your mood, generate optimism, increase your well-being, help you bounce back faster, enhance your self-esteem, make you kinder, improve your social connections, decrease your risk of alcoholism, help you sleep better, help you recover more quickly from illness, boost your immunity, decrease your risk of infections and even help you make more money. The pill has no known side effects. What's more, it's generic and has no copayment! Would you take it?

Yes ❑   No ❑

If you answered yes, here is its secret name: a daily practice of gratitude. Research shows that gratitude can increase your happiness by 25 percent. Gratitude also positively influences your physical health.

Let's explore some ideas to cultivate a more grateful disposition. The following exercises are designed to help you integrate gratitude into your life. Our goal is to lower our gratitude threshold so that we are grateful for little things, sprinkle gratitude multiple times during the day by creating a discipline, and make having grateful thoughts a priority.

Applying Gratitude

Remember: Millions Lack What You Have

Think of anything you have. Millions of people live without those gifts, from the simplest to the most coveted. The table below shows the number of people in the world today who lack the most basic needs for survival.

Need	Number of people without
Safe drinking water	More than 1 billion
Enough food	More than 800 million
Good eyesight	285 million
Good hearing	More than 280 million
Work	More than 200 million
Parents (orphan children)	150 million
A place to live	More than 100 million

The purpose of this awareness is not to feel guilty when you drink water or eat your dinner. It's to feel grateful, realizing each of these is a tremendous gift. Do not delay appreciating the value of these gifts. With gratitude, you'll enjoy these gifts even more. With true gratitude, you find reasons to be thankful instead of waiting for something extraordinary.

It's highly likely that millions of people in the world who are worse off than you and I are, are happier than we are. This is partly because they fully appreciate what they have, even if they don't have much.

Keeping this in mind, let's turn to the next page and find gratitude for an object that I'm sure you haven't appreciated so far.

Change Your Gratitude Threshold

Think about a ripe, juicy pear or other fruit that you recently ate. Did you feel grateful for it?

Yes ❏   No ❏

If you said yes and feel good about your gratitude practice, well, that was a trap! This exercise is not to help you feel grateful for the pear. I want you to be grateful for the *stalk* of the pear — the same stalk that you threw away without taking a moment to think about it. Be creative here and make note of reasons to be grateful for the stalk. Use the space provided below.

Wasn't this stalk the precarious support that held the pear during its growth? It provided security and was the umbilical cord that nourished the pear. No stalk, no pear. Can you be grateful to the stalk for making the pear happen? You can cultivate gratitude for what may seem of little immediate value (such as a grocery store clerk).

☺ Try to feel grateful for two people in your life who seem unimportant today. On the next page, list these people and write why you feel grateful for them.

Person	Grateful thoughts

I hope that with this lowered threshold, you will find it easier to be grateful for your loved ones, friends, colleagues and others who mean a lot more to you than a pear's stalk.

Gratitude gives the same happiness, whether you are grateful for little or big things. By lowering your gratitude threshold, you lift your spirits, which gives you more energy to fully live your day.

Find Gratitude Amid Adversity (what went right within what went wrong)

Matthew Henry, an 18th-century Bible scholar, understood the profound value of gratitude. After his purse was robbed, he wrote this in his journal: "Let me be thankful, first because I was never robbed before; second, because although he took my purse, he did not take my life; third, because although he took all I possessed, it was not much; and fourth, because it was I who was robbed, not I who robbed." He taught us how to reinterpret an adverse experience using the virtue of gratitude.

☺ Think of two past adverse situations and reflect on the aspects that could have gone wrong but didn't. On the next page, write about these experiences in the space provided.

Adversity	What went right within what went wrong

Your focus on the right doesn't mean you deny the wrong. It simply preserves your sanity and saves your energy to better fix the wrong. Gratitude doesn't mean everything is hunky-dory, so let's stop worrying and start partying. Gratitude means you have enough blessings, so you can choose to be happy in this moment.

Find Meaning Amid Adversity

On the evening of Aug. 21, 1883, a devastating tornado ripped through Rochester, Minnesota. It caused 37 deaths and more than 200 injuries, destroyed 135 homes, and leveled 10 farms. With no local hospital, a doctor, his two sons and Mother Mary Alfred Moes of the Sisters of St. Francis cared for the patients in a dance hall. They quickly realized that Rochester needed a hospital of its own. The hospital they founded ultimately became Mayo Clinic. If it hadn't been for the tornado, Mayo Clinic might not have been founded.

☺ Most transformations are seeded by adversities. Reflect on your life's adversities. Have they helped you grow? How? Record your thoughts in the space provided on the next page.

Adversities that helped me grow	How

Consider what you've written; can you be — or begin to be — somewhat grateful for your adversities? Don't waste your hurts. Not learning from a mistake is a bigger mistake. Use your hurts as lessons that help you grow. That process starts with gratitude.

🐦 **Food for Thought:** Most transformations are seeded by adversities. 🐦

Make Gratitude a Habit

The goal is to move the mind from thinking about gratitude occasionally to making it second nature. Forming a new habit takes effort. Effort is worthwhile if the outcome is meaningful. However, even the most meaningful ideas gather dust if they don't become part of the routine. Here are a few tips to help you develop a gratitude routine.

▶ **Keep a gratitude journal.** Write in a gratitude journal every day. Be as specific as possible. You don't have to be very elaborate. Turn to the next page for an example.

Today I'm grateful for . . .	Morning jog Hot cup of coffee at work A chat with Billy, who I hadn't seen in months My partner's smile when I came home My computer didn't crash

☺ In the box below, write about what you're grateful for today.

Today I'm grateful for . . .	

▶ ☺ **Create gratitude index cards.** Think about the people you admire. Write on a few index cards the traits or actions that inspire you. Bring your feelings of gratitude for the inspiration they provide you. In the box below, write the name of one person who inspires you and why you are grateful for that person.

Name of person	Why I'm grateful for this person

On a day when you feel down, pick up one or two cards and draw energy from the life of the person on each card.

▶ **Use gratitude cues.** Any new habit needs reminders. If you have struggled to get your kids to clean up their rooms or train your spouse to separate light fabrics from dark when doing the laundry, you know how hard it is to break an old habit. Cues are great reminders to instill a habit. Here are several gratitude cues to try.

- ❩ A collage of pictures of people you love on your bedroom wall where it's the first thing you see when you wake up
- ❩ Gratitude calendar
- ❩ Mondays marked as gratitude day on your weekly schedule
- ❩ Gratitude app
- ❩ Gratitude wrist band
- ❩ Gratitude sticky note

Can you think of additional cues? Write them in the space below.

- ❩ ☺ **Start a gratitude ritual with children.** Practicing gratitude together as a family is an effective way to make it a habit. Before dinner or at bedtime, ask your children to share one experience from the day that they're grateful for.
- ❩ ☺ **Make a gratitude jar.** Keep an empty jar, scratch paper and a pen in an accessible place at home. Ask family members to write one thing that they're grateful for every day on a piece of paper and drop it in the jar. Encourage them to be funny. During dinner or leisure time, take a few of the notes out of the jar and enjoy reading each other's thoughts.

At our daughter Gauri's elementary school, a fourth-grader recently moved from overseas. Coming from an economically challenged part of the world, she seemed particularly chirpy. When Gauri asked the secret of her happiness, she said, "When I play in the yard here, I don't have to worry about glass splinters or thorns, the swings work and don't creak as much, and you have blue sky. Where I come from, there is so much smog that I haven't ever really seen blue sky."

That little girl was noticing things we hadn't appreciated for years. The precious lesson she taught Gauri and me was this: We shouldn't take anything for granted. We should learn to be grateful for little things. We shouldn't lose something or someone to appreciate its true value. We should love the living and not wait to praise them in a memorial service. We'll need to become humble and more mature to develop such gratitude. What's the outcome we seek?

We wish to be equally thankful for the nourishing apple as well as the stalk and the seeds (that we throw away without noticing), which made the apple happen. Eating an orange, we wish to be equally grateful for the flesh and the bitter rind that protects it. We wish to lower our threshold for gratitude so that we can truly treasure our most precious blessings — the wonderful people we live with and meet each day.

With such gratitude, everything around you becomes extraordinary. Albert Einstein describes this beautifully: "There are two ways to live: You can live as if nothing is a miracle; you can live as if everything is a miracle." If we wish to live as if everything is a miracle, you and I need to cultivate greater gratitude. Happiness talks the language of gratitude. The only limit to your happiness is your creativity in finding gratitude, during both sunny and cloudy days.

Plant the tree of gratitude in the garden of your life. It'll grow the fruits of joy for you and everyone around you for generations to come.

TRY THIS TODAY

Start a gratitude ritual, whether it's writing in a gratitude journal, creating gratitude index cards or using gratitude cues, such as marking Mondays as your gratitude day on your calendar or writing *gratitude* on a sticky note to help you remember to take time to be grateful for the gifts in your life.

Compassion

Understanding Compassion

Compassion is sharing others' sorrows as well as joys. The pursuit of compassion will make you happier than the pursuit of happiness will. Let's enhance our happiness by organizing our lives around the virtue of compassion.

Consider these difficult situations and how you would respond to them.

Your niece just got accepted into Harvard, while your son with a learning disability has fallen back three grades. Will you truly feel happy for your niece and celebrate her success?	❑ Yes ❑ No
Your friend Lisa recently separated from her husband after she caught him cheating for the second time this year. All these years, you have secretly envied their happy married life. Will you truly feel sorry for Lisa and try to support her?	❑ Yes ❑ No
Your friend has hit a snag while working on a project critical to his future success. He asks for your help because you worked on a similar project in the past. He has been your competitor since high school and has always been a bit more successful than you have been. Will you help him?	❑ Yes ❑ No

Every time you answered yes, you were practicing compassion.

Compassion is your ability to feel others' feelings, with a desire and effort to help. Compassion decreases suffering, helps those in need and also celebrates together. It is the practice of the golden rule.

Using this definition, write your last two acts of compassion below.

1.
2.

Now answer this question:

Do I feel good about myself when I remember my compassionate acts?	❑ Yes ❑ No

If you said yes, you have already found meaning in your compassion.

Meaning in Compassion

Compassion helps you in many ways. The table below summarizes some benefits of compassion. Check the yes or no boxes if you agree with these thoughts and write your own perspectives about each point in the third column.

Perspective	Agree?	My perspectives
Receiving or giving compassion can make me healthier.	❑ Yes ❑ No	
Receiving or giving compassion can decrease my stress and make me happier.	❑ Yes ❑ No	
Receiving or giving compassion takes my attention away from my own challenges for a moment.	❑ Yes ❑ No	
Kindness is one of the most important traits I seek in my partner.	❑ Yes ❑ No	
Compassion is essential for our survival as a society.	❑ Yes ❑ No	
Compassion is essential for spiritual well-being.	❑ Yes ❑ No	

Every time you answered yes, you voted in favor of compassion.

🍃 **Food for Thought:** Compassion is decreasing suffering, helping those in need and also celebrating together. It is the practice of the golden rule. 🍃

Applying Compassion

Practicing compassion means:

▶ Developing an ability to see others from their perspective
▶ Removing personal barriers to practicing compassion
▶ Making the practice worthwhile

Next, I'll share ways you can bring these ideas together when you practice compassion.

Compassion in Four Steps

You see an unclaimed kitten outside your door. Freezing rain is falling, and temperatures will drop below zero this evening. You aren't a cat person and start sneezing when a cat is around. Nevertheless, after checking with your spouse, you bring the cat into your home. Let's break this kind action into four steps.

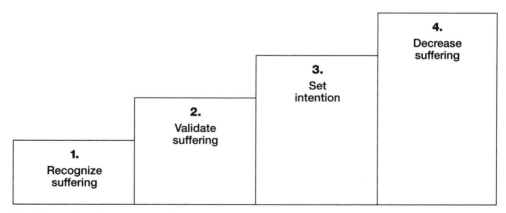

The four steps to compassion

Step 1. Recognize suffering. When you're stuck in your default mode, in the company of your struggles, you seldom recognize others' suffering. Fear is the greatest deterrent to compassion. You have to step outside your mind's wanderings and fears and truly pay attention to the person in front of you. Only then can you understand the challenge from the other person's perspective. In the example of the unclaimed cat, you had a choice to focus either on your sneezes or on the suffering that the cat might have to endure if she stayed outside.

Step 2. Validate suffering. The next step is validating others in your mind. Remaining judgmental and blaming someone for his or her situation hampers your ability to validate suffering. It helps to remember that no one invites suffering. Whenever you can, blame the situation and not the person stuck in it. Spend as little time as you can blaming the person who let the cat loose and instead focus on the cat's suffering.

Step 3. Set intention. Once you cross the hurdle of your judgments and validate the other person, the next step is to recognize that you can actually do something about the situation. You might not be a cat lover and may not want to keep the cat for long, but maybe you can give it shelter for the night.

Even after recognizing and validating someone's suffering, we don't always set the intention because we feel incapable of helping. Sometimes we fear that we might emotionally hurt others or invade their privacy. Most of these fears are overblown. In almost every situation in life, you can do something. Even a few compassionate words can lift a person out of misery. If you offer your help humbly, gracefully and with respect, you'll likely be led in the right direction.

Step 4. Decrease suffering. The primary barriers to tangible actions are: doubting that you can do anything, not knowing or being comfortable with what to do, and fear. To take care of the cat, you'll have to move past the fear that your allergies might flare up. Balancing moral responsibility with appropriate caution is reasonable. If cat exposure gives you life-threatening allergies, then of course it's OK for someone else to keep the cat for the night.

Let's take another look at compassion from the perspective of one of my patients who, without support from family or friends, braved a life-threatening illness that lasted several months. She shared what she would have liked others to have done to help her during her darkest moments. Check the ideas that make sense to you and add other ideas you think may have helped her.

- ❏ Bring her some hot soup.
- ❏ Mow her lawn or shovel her snow.
- ❏ Leave disposable plates and forks for days when she didn't want to wash the dishes.
- ❏ Take her kids to a movie.
- ❏ Offer to take out her garbage.
- ❏ Spend time with her.
- ❏ Take her kids for a sleepover.
- ❏ Walk her dog.
- ❏ Sing her a song.
- ❏ Validate her concerns.
- ❏ Give her an interesting book to read.
- ❏ Your idea _____
- ❏ Your idea _____
- ❏ Your idea _____

All of this can be summed up by a powerful lesson a former colleague once taught me: The most important step to comfort someone is to just show up. You don't have to do miraculous things or say transforming words to help someone. Just show up with an open heart.

Pillars of Compassion
Compassion stands on two strong pillars:

1. Connection
2. Meaning

The more connected you feel with others and the more meaning you find in them, the greater your compassion. Let's address how these two pillars of compassion work.

Connection. How you view your connections with others depends on your interdependence and similarity with others.

In the box below, write some things you can do without help from anyone else.

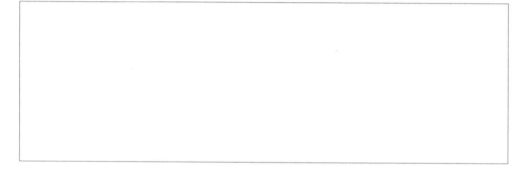

You may have left the box empty or written only one or two things. Just as your heart, liver and kidneys depend on each other (failure of one organ eventually leads to failure of all), we are mutually interdependent. You and I are different wheels on the same cart.

Let's next explore similarities. Think of Kaya, an Eskimo living in the Arctic. He is the father of two children and lives with his wife and elderly parents. Think of some obvious similarities between you and Kaya.

- You and Kaya share 99.9 percent of genes.
- You both have similar biological needs (food, air, water, warmth).
- Your experience of pain, fear, love and joy are identical.
- Kaya is as concerned about his loved ones' safety as you are about yours.
- You both don't want to hurt anyone.
- You both celebrate with food, music and a good time with friends.

Can you think of other ways you and Kaya are similar? Write them below.

```
┌─────────────────────────────────────────────────────────────┐
│                                                               │
│                                                               │
│                                                               │
│                                                               │
│                                                               │
│                                                               │
│                                                               │
│                                                               │
└─────────────────────────────────────────────────────────────┘
```

Research shows that when you find more similarities with others, you feel a stronger connection with them and have greater compassion.

One of the most enjoyable exercises we do in our workshops is to pair up participants in small groups and encourage them to find out what they have in common. Often, in 20 minutes, a group of four or six people can find more than 100 things they all have in common. I almost always find it difficult to end this exercise because everyone gets so immersed in it. Finding what they have in common brings them closer to each other, potentially starting lifelong friendships. If someone annoys you today, think about everything you have in common with that person. It will make you more compassionate.

Meaning. What do you mean when you say that someone means a lot to you? Let's use the three statements below to explain meaning. Read them and choose the one you think will have the greatest impact on you.

1. Flooding kills 20 people on a planet in the Helix Nebula.
2. Flooding kills 20 people in an African village you've never heard of.
3. Flooding kills 20 people in the town where you grew up.

The third statement will affect you the most because you find the people in your town the most meaningful (and connected) to you.

Meaning is related to shared experience and interdependence. I believe that the greater your ability to place yourself in others' shoes and understand them from their perspectives, the more meaningful you find them.

☺ Choose one person in your life and use these ideas to enhance your compassion for that person by finding greater connectedness and meaning.

Name of the person:		
Connectedness		**Meaning** (what makes this person meaningful to me)
Interdependence (how we depend on each other)	**Similarity** (what we have in common)	

Now that you understand some of the essential aspects of compassion, I will share a few exercises for you to try.

Compassion Exercises

Exercise 1: Be compassionate, for you have committed the same mistakes.
Which of these have you secretly desired?

- ❏ Wished that someone's plans would fail
- ❏ Were tempted to do something dishonest
- ❏ Wanted to lie or lied
- ❏ Felt like punching someone in the nose
- ❏ Badmouthed someone more than he or she deserved
- ❏ Fantasized about someone other than your spouse or partner

If you answered yes to any or all of them, know that this is true for all of us. Others are making the same mistakes that you've made or were on the brink of making. They're climbing the same steps that you just did or might. Offering compassionate understanding instead of negative judgment will help them — and you — grow.

Exercise 2: Have you received compassion?
Which of these have you experienced?

❏ Did someone pick me up when I was 6 years old and fell from a bicycle?
❏ Did someone save me when I almost drowned while leaning to swim?
❏ Have I received unexplained kindness from others?
❏ Have I dodged a ticket or two while speeding?
❏ Has someone covered for me in my absence?
❏ Other _____
❏ Other _____
❏ Other _____
❏ Other _____

It's likely that some or all of these may be true for you. By practicing compassion, you are only repaying the debt you owe to the world.

> ✐ **Food for Thought:** By practicing compassion, you are only repaying the debt you owe to the world. ☞

Exercise 3: Have a compassionate heart.
During a community talk, I was heckled by a middle-aged woman who seemed to disagree with everything I said. She was rude and disruptive. We were at a loss as to how to help her. She tested my patience. Eventually, she settled down and allowed me to complete my presentation. At the end of the session, as I was about to leave, she came to talk to me — in tears. Her 16-year-old son had committed suicide two years ago. After losing her son, she had become

averse to all stress management programs. I will never forget the lesson she taught me. Now when I face an unkind person, my first reaction is to ask, *Why is this person suffering? Why is healing not happening here?* These two questions lead me down a completely different path than I would have followed before. I am more easily able to reach the root cause.

☺ Think of a situation in your life in which a person was upset with you. Try to answer these two questions the best you can.

Situation:	
1. Why is this person suffering?	
2. Why is healing not happening here?	

Thoughtfully pursuing the answers to these two questions will lead you to a more compassionate healing and happier path.

Compassion: A Few Last Suggestions
Plan Ahead
Compassion becomes easier when you plan your response in advance. Let me share an example from my clinical practice.

Person and situation	I saw a 35-year-old patient with newly diagnosed breast cancer and an overactive thyroid. I was warned that she was angry with the world. She declined every treatment. When I asked her why, she said she didn't trust doctors. Then she started questioning my competence.
Reflexive response	My reflexive response would have been to disengage from her care, leave her alone to suffer and not invest any energy. I could have even reacted to her, making the problem worse. She faced exactly this response from several health care providers at other facilities.
Compassionate response	Thankfully, I was able to give compassion a chance by delaying judgment and practicing patience. I asked her to tell me her whole story. It was clear that she had good reasons not to trust doctors. She had experienced lack of compassion, incompetence and greed in the past. I validated her experience and shared with her why she shouldn't expect the same disappointments that she had experienced before. Eventually, her distrust turned into trust and she accepted the treatments offered to her.

My compassionate response was only possible because I remembered this: An expression other than love is a call for help. If someone you encounter is upset, he is trying to say he is hurt and needs your help. Your compassion will help much more than your anger will. I can't tell you how many unhappy moments I have avoided since I taught my brain that an expression other than love is almost always a call for help. The formula is:

upset = hurt = call for help

You have a choice to follow one of the two paths listed below.

Event	Your interpretation	Your action	Outcome
Someone is upset.	**Path A:** He is hurt.	This is his call for help.	Compassionate response (healing)
	Path B: He is insulting me.	I need to counterattack.	Aggressive response (hostility)

☺ Although path B is the usual knee-jerk response, path A represents the truth more often. Plan your compassionate response (path A) in the boxes below for someone who frequently gets on your nerves.

Person and situation	
Anticipated current response	
Planned compassionate response	

Just as you plan your trips weeks or months ahead, plan your mind's travel into compassion. Planning ahead will make your compassionate response much easier.

Each time I have forgotten to give compassion a chance, I have regretted it. I'm now committed to compassion for the rest of my life. I know I will fail, but I also know that this commitment will make me and others happier. Consider making the same commitment to yourself.

Approach Those Who Are Suffering

We all have a compassionate core but often can't express our compassion as much as we want to. Identify your barriers to compassion on the next page.

❏ I'm too shy or uncomfortable.
❏ I'm not sure if I'll upset others.
❏ I'm not sure if they need my help.
❏ I'm not sure what I can do.
❏ I'm not sure that what I do will help.
❏ Other _____
❏ Other _____

You have a choice: Remain in your shell or share moments of compassion. When you look back at life, you're more likely to regret not taking action than taking a compassionate action, even if the compassionate action feels a little awkward. Once you see that most people are struggling with their vulnerable selves, compassion will naturally follow. Almost everyone is open to well-meaning compassion. No patient has ever complained of getting too many flowers while in the hospital.

Consider Random Acts of Kindness
☺ A very effective way to taste the joy of compassion is to do random acts of kindness. Which of these are you comfortable doing?

❏ Paying for a stranger's toll.
❏ Letting someone go ahead of me in the checkout line.
❏ Visiting nursing home residents and spending time with them.
❏ Volunteering at a free medical clinic.
❏ Joining a group to adopt a highway.
❏ Praying for a stranger.
❏ Other _____
❏ Other _____

Your random act of kindness can give you greater happiness than some of the most expensive gifts. As a bonus, each random act of kindness is a seed that can start a phenomenon.

Don't Forget Self-Compassion

As a grown-up, you may have received many different expressions of "I love you" and "I hate you." Estimate the number of I-love-you and I-hate-you expressions you've received that are stuck in your heart.

If you're like the rest of us, of all the feedback you receive, you focus on the comments that rate you the lowest. This instinct won't allow you to be happy with yourself. When you aren't compassionate to yourself, you can't be compassionate to others.

Let's try an alternative. Do you have people in your life who love you unconditionally? If yes, write their names below.

These people believe that you mean well. Those who trust your intentions won't negatively judge your each action. With this in mind, practice self-compassion with these ideas.

☺ 1. Look at yourself through the eyes of the person who believes in you, loves you unconditionally and knows that you carry good intentions.
☺ 2. Evaluate yourself by your intentions, not the outcome of your actions.

You can never assure a certain outcome, but your intentions are always in your control.

Finally: Do Not Postpone Loving Yourself

Being compassionate to yourself is the beginning of your journey toward having compassion for the world. Be compassionate to yourself so that you can be your lifelong friend. Self-compassion is neither enabling nor arrogance. Self-compassion is humble integration of your imperfections into your view of the self, with an eye toward growth and improvement. Your self-compassion is essential to sustained happiness. It'll help you accept yourself as you are — our next step in this journey.

TRY THIS TODAY

When you encounter someone who is upset, remember: An expression other than love is a call for help. Respond with compassion rather than anger or judgment.

Acceptance

Understanding Acceptance

We live with countless unknowns. Who created our universe and why? How much suffering is in store for us? And the question of greatest immediate concern — how long will you live — can't be definitively answered. You can either allow yourself to be frazzled by these uncertainties and become unhappy or invite the wisdom of acceptance.

Acceptance is choosing to see the world in its broadest possible context. Let's start by answering these questions.

Will mourning the snowman prevent it from melting?	❏ Yes ❏ No
Can I keep anyone alive until eternity?	❏ Yes ❏ No
Can both players win a game of tennis?	❏ Yes ❏ No
Can a caterpillar keep its 16 legs as it becomes a butterfly?	❏ Yes ❏ No
Can I get taller after I reach my adult height?	❏ Yes ❏ No
Can I change all of my genes?	❏ Yes ❏ No
Can I choose the country of my birth?	❏ Yes ❏ No
Can I choose my biological parents?	❏ Yes ❏ No

I'm sure that by answering these questions, you see that there are many aspects of your life that you can't change. Mourning won't prevent a snowman from melting; you don't get to choose your parents or country of birth.

The less you struggle with the things you can't change, the more energy you save for the things that you can. A more useful response is to accept what you can't change, find meaning in it and make the best of the situation.

Let's look at some aspects of life that *are* in your control, at least to some extent.

Can I improve my driving skills?	❑ Yes ❑ No
Can I lower my cholesterol?	❑ Yes ❑ No
Can I lose weight?	❑ Yes ❑ No
Can I improve my emotional well-being?	❑ Yes ❑ No
Can I exercise on most days?	❑ Yes ❑ No
Can I improve my relationships?	❑ Yes ❑ No
Can I become more expressive in love?	❑ Yes ❑ No

Perhaps you checked yes for most of these questions.

So how should you approach the things that can be changed but are still a work in progress? Consider these seven ideas.

1. Recognize the aspects that can be changed.
2. Recognize the aspects that need to be changed.
3. Find ways to institute the change.
4. Until the change happens, accept things as they are.
5. Don't let this acceptance weaken your change efforts.
6. Recognize that once the desired change happens, you may want further change (the change may not be enough to satisfy you).
7. Understand that despite all your efforts, the change may never happen.

Further, once the change happens, your mind will most likely shift its focus on something else you wish to change.

The following words offer one way to express the balance between the desire to want to change others yet accept them as they are: You are perfect as you are, but you can be better. This statement may sound like a contradiction; acceptance, indeed, is a paradox. It's keeping the faith yet not closing your eyes to the facts. It's finding contentment as you strive to progress. Both are necessary: You need contentment so that you don't fight yourself and are peaceful and happy, and you need to strive so that you continue to grow. Enjoying the good, being grateful for it, even as you try to improve, is an optimal blend to help you savor your success and continue to progress at the same time.

> ✒ **Food for Thought:** Acceptance is keeping the faith yet not closing your eyes to the facts. It's finding contentment as you strive to progress. ✒

Acceptance, then, is a state of balance. It means investing greater energy in the process rather than fretting about the outcome. Acceptance is playing the hand you have. It's creatively working with *what is*. Acceptance is being able to shift your focus depending on life's changing circumstances. Enjoy making your snowman, but when the sun shines bright, give your snowman a hug and wave goodbye.

Meaning in Acceptance

Acceptance helps you dance with life rather than feel you are being pushed around. Research shows that acceptance saves energy, stops your fight with the self, helps you engage with what you can control, directs your focus on savoring the moment rather than trying to make it better, and helps improve many medical conditions. For example, acceptance can help improve diabetes management; help soldiers cope with stress; relieve depressive or anxiety symptoms; improve quality of life and satisfaction with life; help assault victims cope; relieve marijuana dependence; ease chronic pain; improve marital satisfaction; relieve tinnitus; ease drug refractory seizures; alleviate skin picking, compulsive hair pulling, obsessive compulsive disorder, heart-related symptoms, chronic pain and psychosis; and aid in smoking cessation.

Next, we'll explore a few ways to invite acceptance into your life.

Applying Acceptance

Allow me to return to silliness in my discussion of the practice of acceptance. Say you're driving on a highway. Suddenly, the engine oil light turns on. How will you respond?

- ❏ I break the light.
- ❏ I ignore the light.
- ❏ I take my car to the repair shop.

You might choose the first two options, but they won't help you and may be expensive in the long run. Your decision to take the car to the repair shop, on the other hand, offers two key components:

1. **Objectivity** — your ability to see things as they are, not as you prefer them to be.
2. **Willingness** — your willingness to engage with the imperfect or undesirable.

Practicing acceptance requires both objectivity and willingness. Acceptance is practiced in two main domains: people and situations.

1. Acceptance of people (others and self)	2. Acceptance of situations
▶ Be grateful for what is right. ▶ Find meaning in what seems wrong. ▶ Find the context in what seems wrong. ▶ Is it really wrong? ▶ Just accept.	▶ Did I create everything good that has happened in my life? ▶ What appears bad today may seem different tomorrow. ▶ A step backward is often a move forward. ▶ I stop enjoying what I'm trying to improve. ▶ Run my lap and pass the baton. ▶ Accept the inevitability of transience. ▶ Will it matter five years from now? ▶ What percent of life is right versus wrong?

Let's discuss several ways you can improve your acceptance of people and situations.

Acceptance of People

Be grateful for what is right. Consider this situation. You were asked to complete a difficult and involved project within a week. You canceled your planned vacation, dodged your children's boos and immersed yourself in work. After several all-nighters, finally you meet the Friday deadline. Saturday morning, your boss calls you, and his first curt comment is, "Tim, you forgot to number the pages. Remember that next time." Describe your feelings.

Where do you think your boss went wrong? Didn't he focus only on what wasn't right? If he had appreciation and gratitude for all that went right, he would have accepted this minor imperfection and not spoiled your weekend. The message here is to not focus only on blemishes. Express gratitude for what is right before you mention what could be improved.

Find meaning in what seems wrong. Here's another situation to consider. Bob struggles with attention deficit. He is very successful in business, is a great provider and is kind. He has started several successful companies but can't stick with any of them for long. He gets distracted easily. He frequently interrupts you during conversations. Over the years, he has supported his family very well, but he isn't fun to live with because he's so scattered. Going on a vacation with him is a nightmare. He refuses to see the doctor for his attention issues. Can you find some meaning in Bob's attention deficit? Write your ideas in the space below.

Is it possible that Bob's attention deficit actually helped him become a successful businessman? In turn, could his attention deficit have offered his family financial security?

☺ In the space provided below, think of an imperfection in your loved one and try to find meaning in it.

Imperfection	Meaning

Adversity becomes a learning opportunity when you find meaning in it.

Find the context for what seems wrong. You don't find your girlfriend Cindy fun or adventurous anymore. She hates candlelight dinners and hiking in exotic places. Her bedroom at night is as bright as daylight. You're thinking about moving on. But yesterday you learned that two years ago Cindy was grabbed by someone in a dark bathroom. She barely escaped an assault. Since then, she has avoided dark places. How will this knowledge change your attitude toward Cindy?

Won't you become more compassionate and understanding? Judging a person out of context is the same as calling a book uninteresting after reading a random page. Finding the right context in what seems wrong makes you more accepting.

🕊 **Food for Thought:** Adversity becomes a learning opportunity when you find meaning in it. 🕊

☺ List one or two of your loved one's imperfections and try to find rational context.

Imperfection	Rational context

What can you do if you can't find a rational context? Ask yourself, *Is it really wrong?*

Ask yourself, *Is it really wrong?* We're all different. A rainbow has seven colors; each color has its place. What if you took one away? The world would be bland if we all become boringly similar.

Do you have any benign quirks? Do your loved ones have quirks? Try to see them as neither right nor wrong, just different.

List a few attributes that make someone close to you different from you. For example, you might load the dishwasher like a jewelry box, while he stuffs it like garbage can. Without focusing on meaning or rational context, try to see him as just different. He is different, and it's OK.

My style	My loved one's style

☺ Pick one attribute from the list of differences between you and your loved one and accept it for the next week. Grow your list in the following weeks.

Just accept. Finally, you have a list of behaviors that seem clearly annoying and have no rational context. Someone cuts you off on the road, a close friend forgets your wedding anniversary, your spouse forgets to start the dishwasher, a colleague sends an email with a nasty virus that infects your hard drive — the list of annoyances can be long. You didn't invite them, but they are right on your doorstep. You have a choice: Give them energy by reacting to them, or deal with them as best as you can by keeping an attitude of acceptance. Accept because it is a better idea and will save you energy and grief in the long run.

Acceptance of Situations

Did you create everything good that has happened in your life? Which of the following gifts or blessings have you enjoyed so far?

- ❏ I was born with a healthy body.
- ❏ I was raised by kind parents.
- ❏ I grew up in a neighborhood with low crime.
- ❏ I received a good education.
- ❏ I was able to pursue the career of my choice.
- ❏ I am blessed with healthy children.

Many of these gifts are a product of where you were born and to whom — variables entirely out of your control. Just as you can't will everything to be good, you can't prevent everything bad. The only choice is to accept that both the desirable and the undesirable will be part of your life's menu. You choose to play the hand you have because the only other choice is not to play.

What appears bad today may seem different tomorrow. I have no doubt that some of life's minor annoyances have saved my life. Our minds confuse good for pleasant. The reality is that many times what is pleasant in the short term could be hurtful in the long term and vice versa. I often ask workshop participants, *Have your setbacks seeded potential future growth?* More than 80 percent say yes. Sometimes blessings pour into your life as unanswered prayers. One man shared a story with me. In the 1960s, he was a bartender on the West Coast. He worked long hours for low pay. On March 1, 1964, at the end of a hectic day, he was planning a trip to Lake Tahoe, Nevada, for weekend fun, but he missed his flight. He was angry and disappointed. The next morning, he woke up to catastrophic news: The flight he had planned to take crashed because of a snowstorm, killing all 85 people on board. He lost several of his buddies in the tragic accident.

Can you think of ways that adversities or annoyances have helped you grow?

Adversity / Annoyance	How it helped my growth

A step back often is a move forward. Say you climb a mountain to the top. Which of the following is a more realistic path?

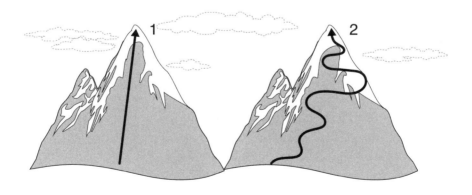

Isn't it image No. 2? Scaling a mountain doesn't ever take a straight path. You climb a few steps and then have to move sideways or even go down a bit to find the right terrain. If you don't follow the longer route, you might slip back to where you started, or worse, get hurt. A step back often is a move forward.

☺ Think about a situation in your life in which a step back actually was a move forward.

🕊 **Food for Thought:** A step back often is a move forward. 🕊

You stop enjoying what you're trying to improve. Have you come across people who can't be pleased no matter what? If yes, why do you think they're so tough to please? Share your thoughts in the box below.

```
┌─────────────────────────────────────────────────────────┐
│                                                           │
│                                                           │
│                                                           │
│                                                           │
│                                                           │
│                                                           │
│                                                           │
│                                                           │
└─────────────────────────────────────────────────────────┘
```

I think they're trying to improve everything and everyone. When seeing a lovely sunset, you might hear them say, "Honey, that sunset looks great. But a little more pink there would have been nicer!" Or, "That baby looks so cute! But her nose is so much like my mother-in-law's!" I hope these are exaggerations.

Remember to balance the urge to improve with appreciation of how good it already is. You stop enjoying what you strive to improve. Not everything needs to be improved and certainly not by you. Experience more, evaluate less.

☺ Pick one upcoming activity, such as a party, a trip or another event. Choose to experience it as it is with a commitment to being patient and nonjudgmental.

🕊 **Food for Thought:** You stop enjoying what you strive to improve. Experience more, evaluate less. Balance the urge to improve with appreciation of how good it already is. 🕊

Run your lap and pass the baton. The relay race is a popular event at the Olympics. Four athletes team up, each taking a turn to run a quarter of the race. The first athlete passes the baton to the second, the second passes it to the third, and the third passes it to the fourth. The fourth runner finishes the race.

What if one day, the fastest runner in the team decides that he will run all the laps? Will it help his team win? The answer is no, because the rules of the game require that all four runners participate equally. The race is about teamwork, coordination and multiple members with talents.

Remember this metaphor when you try to motivate others to change. You can only run your lap. Once you pass the baton to the next person, it's up to that person and his or her effort, motivation and luck. No matter your desire, you can't influence all that.

Accept that transience is inevitable. It's not just the milk carton that comes with an expiration date. We all do. This is called transience. An average person lives about 30,000 days. A hundred years from now, almost everyone living today will be no more. You and I will be long gone. That's the hard truth.

What is your state of mind right now with respect to transience?

❑ I can't accept transience.
❑ I can accept transience, but with resignation.
❑ I fully accept transience.
❑ I don't think about transience.

Continuing to fight with transience generates fear and postpones joy. Accepting transience, on the other hand, offers many benefits. It decreases your fear, saves you energy and inspires you to engage more deeply with life. You have a choice: Fight with transience and remain unhappy, or accept transience and find greater peace.

You may say, *Life is good right now. I am healthy, have good relationships and feel financially secure. Why think about transience and invite sadness?*

I believe there is a good reason. When you realize that you have only a few thousand evenings left with your loved ones, you'll become kinder. You won't say, *Why should I fully live this moment? There will always be a tomorrow.* When you recognize that you are a transient traveler on this planet, you'll take the more scenic route. You'll have fewer regrets if you're present for the present.

I've seen several patients with serious illnesses have the best time of their lives in their last six months. This is because once they realized and accepted their transience, they made kindness and savoring each moment a priority, in favor of letting their minds wander. Each entire day became a flow experience, with their brains in the focused mode. You can learn from their wisdom and do all of this, too. This will make you much happier.

> ✍ **Food for Thought:** When you recognize that you are a transient traveler on this planet, you'll take the more scenic route. ✍

Ask yourself, *Will it matter five years from now?* Which of the following has happened to you in the last five to 10 years?

❏ I received a nasty email.
❏ I got a parking or speeding ticket.
❏ I was treated rudely or unfairly.
❏ Someone I care about ignored me.
❏ I lost money in an investment.
❏ I had to deal with a lazy or negligent person.
❏ Other similarly unpleasant experiences _____
_____
_____

I have experienced all of these in the last 10 years. Earlier in my life, any of these events would have ruined my day. But now I try my best to choose a different response. I zoom out of the experience. I try to look at it from a broader context. By zooming out, what's unpleasant starts to look small and loses its power. The key question I ask myself in these situations is this: *Will it matter five years from now?*

Ask yourself, *Which of these experiences still stew in my mind every day?* If none do, then remember this pearl when you experience adversity again: If it won't matter five years from now, I won't let it matter today.

You can't prevent all adversities or unhealthy thoughts related to them. But you can choose not to allow those thoughts to find a home in your being. You can choose to be a happier person and make happiness a habit.

☺ Commit to this today: Try to broaden your acceptance of imperfections. Just for today, don't let anything that won't matter five years from now matter.

What percent of your life is right versus wrong? Scan the hard drive of your brain and take a look at your entire life. Then answer this question.

What percent of my life is right?
❑ Less than 50 percent
❑ 51 to 75 percent
❑ 76 to 90 percent
❑ More than 90 percent

Most people choose 76 to 90 percent or more than 90 percent. If this is the reality, why aren't we as happy as we can or should be? I think it's because of our tendency to focus on imperfections. It's also because the bad leaves a more intense and lasting imprint than the good. Recognize this quirk in your mind and overcome it by cultivating greater gratitude. Gratitude at its deepest level leads to acceptance.

When you go out on a sunny day, you apply sunscreen so that you won't get a sunburn. Sunscreen allows you to enjoy the day without getting hurt by damaging UV rays. Acceptance is like sunscreen. It allows you to engage with life by helping you adapt to its finiteness, uncertainty and lack of control.

🕊 **Food for Thought:** Acceptance is like sunscreen. It allows you to engage with life by helping you adapt to its finiteness, uncertainty and lack of control. 🕊

Acceptance: Next Steps

At the beginning of this section, I brought up two aspects of life: the changeable and the unchangeable. Let's apply the ideas we've discussed to these aspects. Not all ideas will apply to every situation. Remember the example of the melting snowman? Use what you know about acceptance to reframe other aspects of your life. Feel free to tackle one aspect at a time and come back to others over the next few weeks.

☺ Next, try to reframe the aspects of your life that you can change with one or more of the ideas on the next two pages. Not all the ideas will apply.

I hope this gives you useful insight into the theory and practice of acceptance. Acceptance isn't easy and will be the work of a lifetime, but it's truly worth the effort. It'll help you find greater happiness on your journey to find life's highest meaning.

TRY THIS TODAY

The next time something unexpected happens to you that you can't change, think of how you can make the best of the situation or find meaning in it.

Unchangeable:

▶ Accept that these situations or people can't be changed.
▶ Accept them as they are.
▶ Find meaning in them.
▶ Make the best of the situation as it is.

Aspect of Life	Accepting thoughts
The snowman will melt.	The snow that the snowman is made of melts; that's just the way it is. Joy is in togetherness, not in the snowman lasting forever. Enjoy the snowman while it lasts. When the snowman melts, focus on the warmth of the sun instead of mourning the snowman.
We are all finite.	
Both tennis players can't win.	
A caterpillar loses its legs as it becomes a butterfly.	
You can't get taller after you reach your adult height.	
You can't change all your genes.	
You can't choose the country of your birth.	
You can't choose your biological parents.	

Changeable:

▶ Recognize the aspects that can be changed.
▶ Recognize the aspects that need to be changed.
▶ Find ways to make the change happen.
▶ Until the change happens, accept what is.
▶ Don't let this acceptance weaken your change efforts.
▶ Recognize that once the desired change happens, it may not be enough to satisfy you.
▶ Recognize that despite all of your efforts, the change may not happen.

Aspect of Life	Accepting thoughts
I can improve my driving skills.	My driving isn't too bad, but it could be better. I shouldn't talk on the phone while driving. I should pay more attention to the traffic. I should make enough time for my commute. I can always keep improving my driving skills.
I can lower my cholesterol.	
I can lose weight.	
I can improve my emotional well-being.	
I can start exercising.	
I can improve my relationships.	
I can become more expressive in love.	

Meaning

Understanding Meaning

Children and Socrates have one thing in common: They ask lots of "why" questions. Here is one example of a conversation about "why" that I had with a third-grader.

Third-grader: "Why should I drink milk?"
Me: "So you'll become strong."
Third-grader: "Why should I become strong?"
Me: "So you'll become a big girl."
Third-grader: "Why should I become a big girl?"
Me: "So you can do big things."
Third-grader: "Why should I do big things?"
Me: "So you help others."
Third-grader: "Why should I help others?"
Me: "So you make them happy."
Third-grader: "Why should I make them happy?" . . .

Most of these chains converge to incrementally higher meaning.

Let's try to understand meaning through these three key questions:

1. Who am I?
2. Why am I here?
3. What is this world?

The search for meaning is like walking into dense fog. You see only the next 10 feet. However, as you walk this distance, you start seeing the next 10 feet, and so on.

The answers I suggest for these three questions are placeholders. I have no doubt that as you course through life choosing to learn from it that the fog will clear, and you'll discover better answers.

Who Am I?

Imagine you have to write a short essay about yourself. What would you write?

Perhaps you talked about your relationships, work, hobbies, country and faith.

What if you had to tell the citizens in the Helix Nebula about yourself? These beings are 650 light years away. They know nothing about our solar system. They don't even know what a man is. Your relationships, country, race, work, faith — none of these have any meaning for them. What would you say? (I made a smaller box this time because you might not have as much to say.)

I think that two things transcend age, race, gender, country, religion, and even our planet and solar system: service and love. You and I are agents of service and love. Everything we do fits in these two words.

The specifics about who you are and what you do are the means; service and love are the meaning. All your means converge to this meaning. Your means change, but meaning remains the same. As long as you can be of service and love, you are paying back nature for its gifts. Your bucket is of service and love; the individual roles you play are the candies in the bucket.

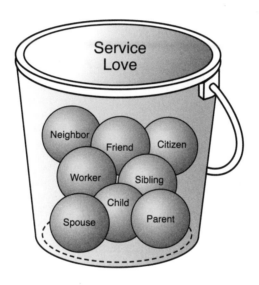

🕊 **Food for Thought:** Two things transcend age, race, gender, country, religion, and even our planet and solar system: service and love. 🕊

Why Am I Here?

We have complex lives with multiple relationships and priorities that are constantly changing. Write your thoughts about what meaningful things you do or hope to do for others in the space provided on the next page.

For my loved ones	
For my friends	
For my neighbors	
For my co-workers	
For my customers and clients	
For others	

Can you tie all the themes together as we just did in the "Who am I" exercise?

One simple way: You're here to make your corner of the world a little happier and kinder than you found it. Adopt a little corner of the world and become its happiness officer.

Consider this world to be a giant canvas. You're given a small corner to paint. You have your brush and paints. Try to draw as lovely a mural as you can, keeping the hope that your work will inspire others, both today and tomorrow, to paint their world the best they can. Charged with this meaning, each day will be one well-lived.

What Is This World?

How old were you when you went to kindergarten? A lot has changed since then. If you can, take a look at your kindergarten picture. How innocent (and ignorant) you were at that time.

All of these years, on most days, you have breathed approximately 20,000 breaths, and your heart has danced 100,000 beats. Breath and heartbeat are the engines that support your brain so that it can do wonderful things and think wonderful thoughts.

What has your brain been doing all this time, in addition to keeping you safe? Learning. Every day your brain changes a bit, depending on your experiences and the new information you present to it.

The world is what you make of it. In kindergarten, it was all play (except for some timeouts). Then, responsibilities, hurts, tests and relationships arrived. All of these have provided you the opportunity to learn. Isn't the world a giant school of learning?

Here is a partial list of the reasons I look at the world as a giant school of learning. Check the items you agree with.

❏ This belief can help me handle adversity better, because I see an adverse experience as an opportunity to learn.
❏ It can help me become wiser, because I am on the lookout for lessons.
❏ It can help me remain humble, because I know I am always a student.
❏ It can help me look forward to life, because I stop running away from my vulnerabilities.
❏ Other _____
❏ Other _____
❏ Other _____

To summarize the three questions:

Who am I?	An agent of service and love.
Why am I here?	To make your part of the world happier and kinder.
What is this world?	A giant school of learning.

Most of your meaning plays out in three areas: relationships, work and spirituality. Let's look at each individually.

Relationships

I'm sure you have someone in your life whom you value more than a trillion dollars. You have the same value — you are priceless. The most important asset of this world is people — you and everyone related or unrelated to you. (I believe everyone in the world is related to you and me.) NASA's mission control celebrated the splashdown of Apollo 13 crew on April 17, 1970, despite the failure of the mission to land on the moon. Failure was less important than NASA's ability to bring the astronauts back safely.

I have posed the following question to many people: What would you do if you knew you had only one minute left in this world? The two most common answers are:

▶ I would call and tell my loved ones how much I love them.
▶ I would pray.

How would you answer this question? Write your answer below.

What would I do if I had only one minute left in this world?	

Bronnie Ware, an Australian palliative care nurse, asked people in the last 12 weeks of their lives to share their top regrets. Three of the top five were related to relationships:

1. I wish I hadn't worked so hard (and missed my children's youth and my partner's companionship).
2. I wish I'd had the courage to express my feelings.
3. I wish I'd stayed in touch with my friends.

Another important regret was, *I wish I had let myself be happier.* Many people regretted not knowing that happiness was a choice. They remained stuck in their old patterns.

As you can see, relationships are very important to our happiness. In a world in which we have more "online followers" than we can ever keep up with, how do we know which members are the most meaningful of our tribe?

Here is a test. Imagine you won $100 million in a lottery. Think about the people who would fulfill these two criteria:

1. They will be truly happy for you.
2. They won't expect a dime.

These are the people who are members of your inner circle. They wish the best for you and have no selfish motives. Let's make a list of the people closest to you who would pass this test.

Member name	Relationship	When I last contacted this person

Don't be surprised if you only have one or two members who meet these criteria. They may not be your blood relatives, and you may not have contacted them in a while. In Week 8, I will present a few ideas to help you seed and feed your relationships with these wonderful people.

Work

You serve the world by your work. Your work is your gift to society. You make the world better and happier with what you do.

Work encompasses many aspects. You may be a business executive, homemaker, janitor, politician, priest, child care provider, teacher, baby-sitting grandma — and all of these roles contribute positively to society. The tangible returns from society might be different, depending on how society views what you do. Trading spices may have made you a millionaire in the first part of the second millennium, while professional acting or playing soccer wouldn't have taken you far. In modern times, how society values these roles has changed.

The lesson here is this: Try not to value what you do only by how many dollars you make. Value it based on its meaning to you and your perception of whether you make the world kinder and happier by what you do.

> ✍ **Food for Thought:** Try not to value what you do only by how many dollars you make. ☙

Let's see how you look at your work. If you can, select only one choice.

❏ Work is nothing but a nuisance.
❏ It's a heavy chore.
❏ Work just pays my bills.
❏ It's a duty.
❏ My work is my passion.
❏ I am privileged to do what I do.
❏ My work is my calling.
❏ My work is my prayer.

The more demand-resource imbalance, lack of control and lack of meaning you feel you have in your life, the more likely you will see your work as a nuisance or a chore. Later in this section, I'll offer a few ideas to help you experience your work as passion, privilege, calling and prayer.

Spirituality

Spirituality has as many definitions as the number of people defining it. It boils down to what you consider sacred, how you treat others and beliefs that provide you a secure framework for living. Let's take an inventory of what you consider spiritual:

❑ Tending to nature
❑ Meaningful work
❑ Selfless service
❑ Nurturing relationships
❑ The present moment
❑ Faith in God
❑ Practicing my faith (prayer, observances, rituals)
❑ Practicing the principles of my faith (gratitude, compassion, acceptance, forgiveness)
❑ Other _____
❑ Other _____
❑ Other _____

All of these can be considered spiritual. Whenever you find life and this world sacred and treat it gracefully and with honor, you experience and practice spirituality. Living an ethical, moral life is the greatest spiritual practice.

> 🕊 **Food for Thought:** Living an ethical, moral life
> is the greatest spiritual practice. 🕊

Meaning in Meaning

Every second, five babies are born. I have spent countless hours in the delivery room, both as a provider and a parent. The sound everyone craves to hear as soon as the baby is born is a loud cry. To mom and dad and the medical staff, a newborn's loud cry is a more pleasant and meaningful sound than the song of the sweetest canary.

Fast-forward three months. It's 2 a.m. and you are tired, with puffy eyes from lack of sleep. But your little one has a soiled diaper and is hungry. She is crying, too — at the top of her lungs. How does her crying sound now? Worse than a hammer hitting you on your head, right? It's the same cry, but what has changed is its meaning.

Meaning changes everything. A positive meaning makes adversity worthwhile; it can even infuse adversity with happiness. Being able to find positive meaning is the hallmark of resilience. No wonder research shows that being able to find meaning helps you be healthier, happier and more focused — with better ability to cope; lower anxiety, depression and stress; improved quality of life; less anger; greater success; and better relationships.

☺ The more you think of higher meaning, particularly in an adverse situation, the more productive and happier your life will be. Let's see if you can enhance the meaning for one or two unpleasant situations in your life. Ask yourself, *Did adversity prevent something worse? Did adversity help you grow?*

Adversity	Meaning

Viktor Frankl's words ring true here: "Suffering ceases to be suffering at the moment it finds a meaning."

Applying Meaning

The ideas that follow reflect my understanding related to the three questions — Who am I? Why do I exist? What is this world? — in the three domains: relationships, work and spirituality. Here I focus on finding greater meaning in work and spirituality. Relationships are covered in Week 8.

At Work

Work as if everyone you serve is your family. I trained alongside a brilliant clinician in India who is the most gifted and conscientious doctor I have ever met. His simple secret was this: Treat every patient as if he or she is your close relative.

Connection brings compassion and compassion helps with conscience, which, in turn, influences attention and competence. I have never met anyone who was compassionate yet incompetent.

☺ Cultivating compassion provides a path to competence. Let's see if you can apply this to your life.

What is the nature of my work?	
Who am I serving?	
Can I consider my customers my relatives? What relationship can I think of?	
If I think I'm serving my relatives through my work, do I think that belief might enhance my work? How and why?	

Create and innovate as if your children and grandchildren will use your product, which is very likely to be true. If honeybees and ants can practice this simple idea with their little brains, we certainly can. This belief will help you create better products — not just the ones that attract eyeballs and bring you money and success, but something truly meaningful that makes the world kinder and happier.

🕊 **Food for Thought:** Work as if everyone you are serving
is your family. 🕊

Be humble: Worry less about who gets the credit. At every workplace, you can find a few people who have mastered the art of gaming the system. They know precisely how to take the credit. While such people may occasionally succeed, they will not rise to greatness. Research convincingly shows that the greatest leaders have a combination of passion and humility. They don't try to grab the headlines. They find reward in the process — a design perfected, a customer served — and are not driven by success and fame. If you enjoy doing things for others and aren't worried about who gets the credit, you are in for a treat.

Humility is often misunderstood. In your opinion, which of the following ideas accurately illustrate being humble?

❏ Letting others trample me
❏ Having accurate self-awareness (knowing my strengths *and* my weaknesses)
❏ Having deflated self-worth
❏ Being open to new viewpoints
❏ Practicing self-denial
❏ Balancing self with others' needs

If you chose having accurate self-awareness, being open to new viewpoints and balancing self with others' needs, you are right. Humility is low self-focus, not low self-esteem. Humility is a sign of strength, not weakness.

Humble people are open to experience. They are willing to learn from failure and success alike. They don't swell with praise nor do they collapse with critique. They maintain equanimity and feel as comfortable as a leader as they do being a part of the team.

Humility offers several additional advantages. Here are my top three. See if you can add one or two more.

1. Humility provides freedom.	When you are humble, you feel secure and don't carry the burden of maintaining an inflated view of the self. The opposite of being humble is being narcissistic. A narcissist has a damaged sense of self and has to constantly defend the self, which he or she does through pre-emptive strikes at others.
2. Humility and its cousin, kindness, are contagious.	Others catch the humility bug from you. When you are humble and kind, others feel comfortable around you. They find no need to protect their egos because they don't feel threatened. The result: They become humble and kind when they are with you.
3. Humility leads to success.	Self-awareness, other-awareness, self-compassion and other-compassion are the four key components of emotional intelligence. A truly humble person has all of them. Research shows that career success is closely linked to your emotional intelligence and, in turn, your humility.

Humility has one more benefit. Fame flavored with humility creates much less envy. Envy isn't an emotion we talk about much in our society. I believe envy is as destructive as anger. In fact, a lot of rage, hatred and disgust start with envy. Envy crowds the space that rightly belongs to love. Focus on the hard work someone put in, not on the success he got. Focusing on others' hard work and struggles will inspire you, and enjoying others' happiness will make you happier.

The next question is, how can you cultivate greater humility? Here are a few ideas. Check the ones you agree with.

❏ Know my strengths and weaknesses. Accept them.
❏ Be open to critique. Consider myself a lifelong learner, enrolled in a school of life in which I'll always keep learning.
❏ Listen to and try to fully understand others' viewpoints, even ones that don't align with mine.
❏ Include the needs and preferences of others.
❏ Believe in the people who believe in me.

The last point is the most important. Humility comes from a secure sense of who you are. This security comes from the firm conviction that you are loved and accepted for who you are. Ideally, you want this love and acceptance to flow from everyone — your spouse or partner, parents, siblings, friends, colleagues, teachers, neighbors, employers, employees, and the world at large. But if the flow is lacking from some areas, pay greater attention to the sources that are still flowing. Lease the precious space in your brain to only people who are kind and well meaning.

If you don't feel loved by your partner today but feel deeper connection with your friends, parents, children, grandparents, neighbors or colleagues, then anchor your identity in the latter relationships. This will help you nurture healthier self-esteem and provide you with greater peace and happiness. Hopefully, your partner will recover from his or her black hole and develop greater kindness toward you, and then you can anchor your identity in your relationship with him or her.

☙ Food for Thought: If you enjoy doing things for others and aren't worried about who gets the credit, you are in for a treat. ☙

Find your work entertaining. Every day we pay for entertaining experiences: movies, theatre, dance recitals, baseball games. Could work also become as entertaining?

Imagine a day when you stop needing a regular paycheck. Would you continue to work? If so, what would you do if money wasn't an issue? If what you would do is the same or similar to what you do now, then you have the best job in the world.

Let's take it to the next level. Would you work even if you had to pay for it? If you can say yes, then your work indeed is your passion, privilege, calling and prayer.

You and I need a paycheck to support ourselves and our families. But if we can find greater meaning and joy in our work, then it might become as inviting as our favorite source of entertainment. For your work to assume that quality, you have to be willing to make a few compromises.

Be willing to compromise. I look for these seven characteristics in an ideal job. Check the ones that apply to you and note any I have missed.

My job:
- ❑ Challenges me.
- ❑ Provides a path to growth.
- ❑ Gives me a positive meaning.
- ❑ Provides fair compensation.
- ❑ Has predictable expectations.
- ❑ Allows me optimal control.
- ❑ Respects me for who I am.
- ❑ Other _____
- ❑ Other _____
- ❑ Other _____

Recognize that each workplace is dynamic. It has its own personality and several moving parts. All of these ideals are unlikely to be satisfied all the time, so you'll be happier if you're willing to make some compromises.

Ask yourself, *What do I want to do two jobs from now?* If it's precisely what you're doing today, your work is as good as it can be.

No matter what you do, remember that your work indeed has a higher meaning.

☺ Let's try to connect your work with the larger world: your family, company, community, country and planet. Integrating the characteristics we've just listed, describe how you find greater meaning in your work in the exercise below.

How does my work help my family?	
How does my work help my company?*	
How does my work help my community?	
How does my work help my country?	

How does my work help our planet?	

*If you are a homemaker, your family is your company.

On a day when you don't feel optimistic about what you do, think about this higher meaning. It might pull you out of the whirlpool of negativity. It'll help you find your work spiritual.

Spirituality

Understand your own spirituality. Tending to nature, meaningful work, selfless service, nurturing relationships, the present moment, faith in God, practicing your faith and practicing the principles of your faith are all spiritual.

To understand your spirituality, categorize your outlook on each of these aspects in the following three groups.

Spiritual aspect	Totally believe in it	Not so sure	Don't believe in it at all
Tending to nature	❏	❏	❏
Meaningful work	❏	❏	❏
Selfless service	❏	❏	❏
Nurturing relationships	❏	❏	❏
The present moment	❏	❏	❏
Faith in God	❏	❏	❏
Practicing my faith	❏	❏	❏
Practicing the principles of my faith	❏	❏	❏

Carve your spiritual path.

☺ Based on this understanding, can you think of a few ideas to enhance your spirituality? Let's choose three areas that you totally believe in. I'll start by suggesting some ideas related to nature.

Area of spirituality	Ways to enhance my spirituality in this area
Tending to nature	Spend more time in nature. Recycle. Plant trees. Decrease energy consumption. Contribute to charities that care for nature.
Area of spirituality	**Ways to enhance my spirituality in this area**

Anytime you add a selfless element to your endeavors, consider this world and its beings sacred, and focus on doing the greatest good for the greatest numbers, you are having a spiritual experience.

Live life with higher principles. Living a moral, ethical life is the highest spiritual practice. Practicing gratitude, compassion, acceptance and forgiveness is the bedrock of morality. The approach outlined in this book can help you bring them all into your life.

☺ Research shows that we are all susceptible to dishonesty. Try to live one week with total morality. Notice how your thoughts, words and actions driven by conscience provide greater and sustained happiness. Check the ones you feel comfortable committing to and add a few ideas of your own.

This week:
- ❏ I won't make a promise that I don't intend to keep.
- ❏ I will always speak the truth, even for minor issues.
- ❏ I won't use language with double meaning to hide the truth.
- ❏ I will look at others with kind attention.
- ❏ I will not secretly wish harm on anyone.
- ❏ I won't criticize anyone unless I have to.
- ❏ I won't visit unclean websites.
- ❏ I will drive within the speed limit.
- ❏ I will not waste water or other resources.
- ❏ I will be kind to people who depend on me, such as my co-workers and my children.
- ❏ I will speak gently to telemarketers.
- ❏ I won't use any curse words, even in thought.
- ❏ I will accept others' spirituality.
- ❏ _____
- ❏ _____
- ❏ _____
- ❏ _____

Spirituality doesn't create silos. Accepting others is profoundly spiritual.

🖎 **Food for Thought:** Accepting others is profoundly spiritual. 🖎

Meaning: Additional Understandings

On the next page, I'll share with you two additional perspectives on meaning that I've found helpful over the years.

Meaning Is Contextual

What is meaningful to you today may not be meaningful for somebody else. Further, what was meaningful for you yesterday may not mean much to you today. For example, maybe you don't care about your favorite blanket or beating your cousin in a milk-drinking contest anymore. Ask yourself which of the following experiences used to be meaningful to you but aren't anymore.

Experience	Was very meaningful	No longer as meaningful
A visit from the tooth fairy	❏	❏
Leaving carrots for Santa's reindeer	❏	❏
Showing others how high you can jump	❏	❏
Winning in board games	❏	❏
Being told how big a girl or boy you are	❏	❏
Sitting in the front seat of the car	❏	❏
Other	❏	❏
Other	❏	❏
Other	❏	❏
Other	❏	❏

The next time you're annoyed because you feel you were left out or missed an experience, ask yourself, *Is this another minor preference that won't bother me when I grow up emotionally and spiritually?*

Ultimate Meaning Is Difficult to Fully Understand

Our present meaning is in the process and not in the grand finale. The ultimate meaning of life is comprehensible only when you realize what comes before and what follows it. Until that meaning is unveiled, I believe that living each day as an agent of service and love, having a goal to make your world happier and kinder, and knowing that this world is a giant school of learning will provide you with secure meaning. Such meaning will make you happier and more resilient.

I hope you find your life's deepest meaning.

TRY THIS TODAY

Considering the three questions on meaning — Who am I? Why do I exist? What is this world? — think about what gives your life meaning in terms of your relationships, work and spirituality.

Forgiveness

Understanding Forgiveness

Unlike all the other organs of the body, our minds have no natural system for getting rid of waste. Hurts pile up as open files and black holes. Gratitude for what is right, compassion for suffering, accepting imperfections and focusing on life's higher meaning can all soften life's hurts. But there's one cure that can dissolve all hurts for good: forgiveness.

Forgiveness is a voluntary choice. It means that you choose to give up anger and resentment despite knowing and accepting that the misconduct happened. Forgiveness is choosing the higher path and leading a more thoughtful life driven by your principles. Which of these descriptions do you agree with?

Forgiveness is:
- ❏ A willful choice
- ❏ Living by my principles
- ❏ My gift to others
- ❏ Choosing a higher path
- ❏ Practicing kindness
- ❏ Abiding by my family's and culture's values
- ❏ For me

Forgiveness isn't:
- ❏ Forgetting the wrong
- ❏ Allowing a wrong to continue
- ❏ Excusing the wrong
- ❏ Denying the wrong
- ❏ Letting someone harm me
- ❏ Letting go of legal recourse if I have to

Considering these perspectives, do you agree that forgiveness can help you without making you vulnerable?

Meaning in Forgiveness

Anger, holding a grudge and hostility can all lead to anxiety, depression, irritability, disturbed sleep, higher blood pressure, irregular heart rhythm and a higher risk of heart attack.

Forgiveness, on the other hand, has many benefits. By forgiving, you enjoy improved health, save energy, have better relationships and set an example for others, particularly children. Here are just some of the benefits of forgiveness. Check the ones you agree with and add ideas of your own.

- ❏ Forgiveness can enhance my physical health. It can improve blood pressure, lower heart rate and improve immunity.
- ❏ Forgiveness can improve mental and emotional health by promoting better sleep and lowering anxiety, depression and stress level.
- ❏ Forgiveness can improve my relationships.
- ❏ Forgiveness helps me save my energy.
- ❏ Forgiveness helps me to focus better.
- ❏ Forgiveness helps me feel good about myself.
- ❏ Forgiveness helps me live a more spiritual life.
- ❏ Forgiveness can strengthen my faith.
- ❏ Forgiveness can make me happier.
- ❏ Other benefits _____
- ❏ Other benefits _____
- ❏ Other benefits _____

Applying Forgiveness

Forgiveness doesn't come naturally to the human mind. Forgiveness isn't easy. Here are some reasons why it is such a difficult mountain to climb. Check off which ones you agree with and add additional reasons of your own.

- ❏ The world considers forgiveness a sign of weakness.
- ❏ Forgiving a hurt seems unfair.
- ❏ People fear that forgiveness will make them vulnerable.

- ❏ People feel others may not deserve their forgiveness.
- ❏ People feel forgiveness will take away their rights.
- ❏ Thinking about revenge activates the pleasure centers of the brain.
- ❏ Other _____
- ❏ Other _____

Forgiveness is as intentional as exercising. Because planning revenge activates the brain's pleasure centers, you'll have to make considerable effort to forgive. To forgive, you must:

- ▶ Find the person forgivable
- ▶ Become a more effective forgiver
- ▶ Find meaning in forgiveness

Here are five perspectives and nine pearls to start your journey into forgiveness. If you find forgiveness difficult, try thinking of yourself as a conduit for the forgiveness to flow through, instead of seeing yourself as the source of forgiveness. For hurts that seem unforgivable, you may need help from a licensed mental health professional and the company of someone you trust who can walk with you all the way.

5 Perspectives That Lead to Forgiveness

1. Innocence

Imagine you are leaning forward to pick something up from the floor at home. Suddenly, someone rushes into you from the side, holds your cheek with one hand and pulls on it until your face gets scratched. How does this make you feel?

You probably didn't write words such as *ecstatic, blissful* or *joyous*, right?

If you wrote *angry, mad* or *upset*, let me share who that person is. It's your 9-month-old daughter or granddaughter, who crawled up to you with a surge of emotions. Are you still mad?

When you consider that others' actions reflect innocent ignorance, you are more likely to forgive.

> ✒ **Food for Thought:** When you consider that others' actions reflect innocent ignorance, you are more likely to forgive. ✒

2. Connection

It's 7:55 a.m. You have five minutes to scarf down your breakfast because you have to start a conference at 8 a.m. You are swallowing large chunks of food like an alligator does. Suddenly, pain in your mouth makes you cringe. Your lower left wisdom tooth bit the inside of your cheek. You wait for the hurt to subside before you start eating your breakfast again. This time, you eat more slowly than you did before. Should your wisdom tooth ask your cheek for forgiveness? It sounds silly, doesn't it?

It sounds silly because your tooth and cheek are a part of the whole that is you. When you feel connected to and approve of a person, his or her actions seem good. But if you don't approve of or feel connected to someone, even a minor imperfection can be exaggerated.

The more connected you feel, the easier it is to forgive.

3. Self-defense

Once while visiting a friend, I was sitting in a chair, when unknown to me, his Pomeranian dog came and sat under the chair. When I stood up, I accidentally stepped on her tail. She snarled and bit me on the hand. It was clearly a provoked bite. She was acting in self-defense, reacting to my (innocent) assault. While my friend felt guilty, I had no reason to complain.

Most people are trying to protect their vulnerable selves. Their anger reflects their fear; terse words come from personal hurt. If you consider that others are acting in self-defense and you're often caught in collateral damage, it'll be easier to forgive.

4. Misunderstanding

Several years ago, I offered unsolicited financial help to a close friend. Looking back, I see that I shouldn't have done that. He had come from overseas, I presumed he needed the help, and I hurt his ego because of my misjudgment. But I truly didn't mean to hurt him. My friend saw my ignorance as bad intent, and it created a rift in our relationship. He lashed out at me pretty strongly. I think I didn't speak the right words and was misinterpreted.

The lesson I have learned is this: Many slurs that come my way may not be intended. They may reflect ignorant bad judgment. I shouldn't allow misunderstandings to lead to moments of unforgivable hurts.

5. Meaning

When I was starting my research career, I worked on an ambitious proposal to understand the effect of different mental states on the human body's metabolism. My hope was to use the information to develop innovative mind-body approaches. After putting in more than 1,000 hours of work, I submitted the grant proposal, which was reviewed by two experts. One gave it a glowing review, with the highest possible score. The other gave it bad marks, commenting that he didn't quite understand what I wrote and felt unqualified to review it. My proposal wasn't accepted.

I was angry and disappointed. I had to quit that line of work. But it prompted me to move forward in developing a mind-body program. Now when I look back, I feel it was good that my grant wasn't funded. Although I would have gotten to a place similar to where I am today, it would have taken me at least five more years. I have long forgiven the committee and the people involved and actually am grateful to them for saving me from what might have been unnecessary effort.

Once you find meaning in adversity, it becomes much easier to forgive. Hurts can help, and so can forgiveness.

🕊 **Food for Thought:** Once you find meaning in adversity, it becomes much easier to forgive. Hurts can help, and so can forgiveness. 🕊

☺ Let's apply these elements to your life to strengthen your forgiveness muscles. Think of one situation in your life in which you need to forgive. Apply one or more of these five elements to the situation. Ask yourself if inviting this perspective will make you happier.

Situation:		
Element		**Explanation**
1. Innocence	❏	
2. Connection	❏	
3. Self-defense	❏	
4. Misunderstanding	❏	
5. Meaning	❏	

I have found some pearls that have helped me while applying these elements. These pearls can enhance your understanding of forgiveness and help you sustain it over the long term.

Forgiveness: 9 Pearls

I have been privileged to learn from patients who have shared lifetimes of wisdom related to bringing forgiveness into their lives. Here are nine pearls I have found helpful.

1. Forgiveness Is a Lifelong Process

Can you think of a few difficult activities that you can master after one try or certain skills that never fade after you've mastered them?

Activities I can master after one try	Skills that never fade after I've mastered them

You couldn't think of many, could you? Almost every skill you learn needs practice to master it and continuous practice to keep it fresh. Your body needs food and water every day; otherwise, it becomes depleted. Yesterday's sleep won't compensate for today's need. Your lawn needs mowing every few days to keep it tidy.

Similarly, unforgivingness — the inability or unwillingness to forgive — is the mind's instinct. Even if you have forgiven a hurt today, the same hurt will bother your mind tomorrow. Your mind forgets and needs repeated reminders. You'll have to keep forgiving the same issue many times before it becomes permanent.

2. It's OK to Be Selfish in Forgiveness

Do you agree with the following 3 statements?

❏ I can teach a concept only after I have learned it.

❏ My ability to help others emotionally and spiritually depends on my own emotional and spiritual growth.

❏ To better protect others, I have to become stronger.

You have to take care of yourself before you can take care of others. When flying, for example, if the oxygen pressure drops, you should put the oxygen mask first on yourself before helping your child.

People who hurt us often don't seem deserving of our forgiveness. To start the process, it helps to think that the person most helped by your forgiveness is none other than you.

3. Humans Are Fallible

In your life so far, how many people have you personally met who you think:

Trait	Fewer than 5	5 or more
Are truly wise	❏	❏
Are truly compassionate	❏	❏
Always do the right thing	❏	❏
Live for a higher purpose	❏	❏
Almost never have a personal agenda	❏	❏
Have great self-control	❏	❏
Seldom, if ever, get angry	❏	❏
Always use kind words	❏	❏

Always think of others before themselves	❏	❏
Have all of these qualities	❏	❏

Was your list small? Mine is.

Most of us are fallible. We are limited in our judgments, our minds are led astray when we want short-term gratification, and our thinking is dominated by thoughts of self-protection and personal success. All of this comes without our understanding of the collateral damage we cause in the process. This is no one's fault. It's simply a limitation of our minds.

If you consider humans fallible, your expectations will be lower. This will make forgiving others — and yourself — easier.

4. Don't Let the Hurts Stick for Too Long

To make a vegetable soup, you mix vegetables with salt, spices and water and then let them stew. That's what the mind does. An original thought is spiced with exaggerating, generalizing and catastrophizing, and then we let it simmer in our minds. The hurts crowd our minds, leading us to unforgivingness. The final product is often a spiced-up version of what happened.

☺ The key to avoid a hurt from becoming a black hole is to prevent excessive ruminations about it. How? Here are a few ideas to help you reframe your situation. Several of them will remind you of the themes covered under the topic of acceptance. Check the ones that you find compelling and add thoughts of your own.

❏ Focus on what is right in the other person and be grateful for it.
❏ Think about what I would have done if I were in the other person's situation.
❏ Consider that the other person acted out of ignorance or self-defense instead of meaning to harm me.
❏ Realize that no one is perfect, including me. We all make mistakes.
❏ Consider that what may seem to be a significant hurt or loss today may not bother me in a few years. Ask myself, *Will it matter five years from now?*

- ❏ Focus on the possibility that whatever hurt me may have helped me or will help me in the future.
- ❏ Forgive because I want to be kind to myself and others.
- ❏ Other _____
- ❏ Other _____
- ❏ Other _____
- ❏ Other _____

Try not to let the sun set on unresolved anger, particularly when it is related to minor irritations.

> 🕊 **Food for Thought:** Try not to let the sun set on unresolved anger, particularly when it is related to minor irritations. 🕊

5. Don't Wait for Others to Seek Forgiveness

Have you noticed that people who hurt you start avoiding you? If you hurt someone, whether it was by mistake or willfully, did you:

- ❏ Feel embarrassed?
- ❏ Feel angry?
- ❏ Withdraw from that person?
- ❏ Feel sad?
- ❏ Try to blame that person?
- ❏ Avoid talking about that person?
- ❏ Avoid visiting the thought of what happened?
- ❏ Wish it never happened?
- ❏ Want to apologize but weren't able to muster enough courage?
- ❏ Wish the other person would forgive you without your asking?
- ❏ Feel guilty?
- ❏ Other feelings _____
- ❏ Other feelings _____
- ❏ Other feelings _____

If any of this is true for you, it is for others, too. A hit-and-run accident on the road is against the law. But an emotional hit-and-run is very common and not punishable by any court.

Remember that people feel insecure and need tremendous courage to seek an apology. Forgive before others seek forgiveness. If you wait for the other person to call you, it may be a very long wait, perhaps a lifetime.

6. Forgive Gracefully

Imagine that you spilled coffee on your client at a business meeting. What words would you use to describe how it feels to receive forgiveness from that client? Check all that apply.

❏ Really fun
❏ Embarrassing
❏ Awkward
❏ Joyous
❏ Stressful
❏ Relaxing
❏ Delicate
❏ Dreadful
❏ Other feelings _____
❏ Other feelings _____
❏ Other feelings _____

A personal injury is hurtful. Injuring someone else is equally, if not more, hurtful. Most people find it awkward, stressful and sometimes embarrassing to receive forgiveness. It reminds them of their weakness.

Recognize that while internally you will have to forgive the same action multiple times, people don't like to hear that they are forgiven. It's an assault on their egos. It makes them feel vulnerable.

Forgiveness becomes healing when it's gentle, kind and graceful. Your graceful behavior will inspire others to be equally graceful when it's their time to forgive.

7. Time Your Forgiveness

You are 12 years old and want to have a sleepover with your best friend, but you aren't sure your mother will approve. She seems stressed because your little brother has a cold and isn't eating, the laundry isn't done, and she just had an argument with dad that didn't end well. You also haven't finished your homework and forgot your lunch bag at school. Is this a good time to ask for the sleepover?

The point is this: Everything has a right time, including seeking forgiveness. Here are a few ideas to help you choose the right time to ask for forgiveness. Check the ones you agree with and add thoughts of your own.

It's best to ask for forgiveness:

❑ When the other person is in a happy mood
❑ During an introspective or philosophical moment
❑ After you have done a few good things to earn some brownie points
❑ Shortly after delivering good news
❑ As a birthday or anniversary gift
❑ After visiting a church or another holy place
❑ During a season of forgiveness, such as Christmas
❑ When I have thought through how best to make up for my mistake
❑ Other ideas _____
❑ Other ideas _____
❑ Other ideas _____

Using the right words at the right time is a gift; using the right words at the wrong time can create a rift.

8. Forgive in Honor of Someone You Respect

Many of us need an extra push to succeed at forgiveness. That extra push could be honoring someone whose values and legacy you respect. I find forgiveness much easier when I forgive in the name of someone I know is suffering or someone who truly embodies higher values.

9. Pray to Forgive

Faith is a powerful tool that can help forgiveness. Think of it this way: It isn't up to you to forgive. The energy of forgiveness flows from a higher realm, and you are but a channel for that energy. Your job is to not block its flow; allow the energy to course through you. Pray that the person who hurt you finds healing and wisdom, pray that you are able to forgive, and pray that forgiveness helps you and everyone around you grow spiritually.

Forgiveness Exercises

Forgiveness Imagery

Sometimes it helps to add forgiveness to your relaxation practice. Here are two exercises to try.

☺ **Exercise 1:** On a peaceful, sunny day, watch a distant cloud. Collect all of your hurts and place them on that cloud. Watch the cloud float away, taking all of your hurts with it. Practice deep, relaxed breathing with this exercise.

☺ **Exercise 2:** Mentally collect all that you have to forgive in a folder. Keep in mind that the folder is too heavy and toxic for you to handle. Forward this folder to your higher power, the creator or the universe and let that entity deal with it. Consider your job done.

Release of Emotions

An additional helpful tool is to practice emotion-releasing exercises. Here are two exercises to try.

☺ **Exercise 1:** Write a letter to the person you want to forgive. Include all the details about the event and state clearly why you were hurt. End the letter with a few lines addressing your intention to forgive. Read this letter as if the person has already received it. Then shred the letter.

☺ **Exercise 2:** When you're on a beach, write your grievance on the sand close to the shore. Watch the waves wash the words away. Keep that imagery in your mind so that you can relive this experience of forgiveness.

Forgiveness is the ultimate test of your ability to embody higher principles. The hurt of unforgivingness originates from failure in gratitude, compassion, acceptance and higher meaning. The more effectively you can practice the other four principles, the easier it will be for you to forgive.

Although it's challenging, your journey toward forgiveness is truly worth the effort. It can transform the fate of a nation, as did Nelson Mandela, or inspire humanity until eternity, as did Christ's words, "Father forgive them, for they know not what they do."

TRY THIS TODAY

Forgive one person using one of the techniques in this section.

Week 8: Relationships

Weaving deeper and lasting connections within your community is one of your highest priorities and the final key ingredient of emotional resilience. A closely knit community can do wonders for your happiness. Such a community includes the people who nurture you and depend on you to nurture them. These are the people you think of in your morning gratitude exercise, the people you depend on and who support you when life sends a curveball your way. Your community has four concentric circles:

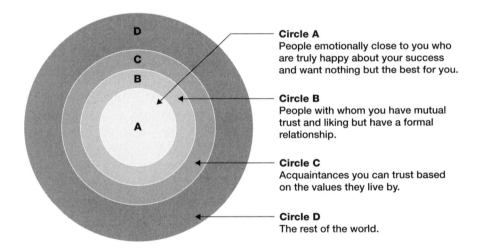

Circle A
People emotionally close to you who are truly happy about your success and want nothing but the best for you.

Circle B
People with whom you have mutual trust and liking but have a formal relationship.

Circle C
Acquaintances you can trust based on the values they live by.

Circle D
The rest of the world.

Cultivating your community, particularly its two innermost circles, isn't much different from cultivating your garden. As you would your garden, nurture your community in three steps: seed, feed and weed.

Seed

Seeding the inner two circles of your community is a process that takes time and energy. Given your busyness, you might overlook this step. Not prioritizing relationships is one of the top regrets people have at the end of their lives.

Your closest, most meaningful relationships are created from two seeds. The first seed is you. The second seed is the special people who are part of your identity and have shared meaning. Find these people by answering these questions.

Question 1: How many people do you know who live by the same or similar ethical principles as you do?

I have repeatedly found that the people most likely to disappoint me are those who have strikingly different moral values. Let's make an inventory of people in your life who you would guess have roughly the same moral values as you do.

Names of people who have moral values similar to mine	
Related to me	
Not related to me	

Question 2: Among the people you listed, how many can you place in one of the circles described below? Write their names in the appropriate boxes.

Circle A: People emotionally close to me who are truly happy about my success and want nothing but the best for me.	
Circle B: People with whom I have mutual admiration, but a formal relationship.	
Circle C: Acquaintances I can trust based on the values they live by.	

☺ Once you fill these circles, make it a priority to connect each week with at least one or two people you feel emotionally close to or admire.

Note that many people in your life won't fit the criteria for circle A and circle B. They may be your co-workers, neighbors, previous friends or even relatives. You'll likely connect with them off and on based on shared short-term meaning. But given that you have a limited amount of energy and time, it'll be worthwhile to invest most of your efforts connecting with people who have shared moral values and who you trust want what's best for you.

Feed

Once you have identified the people you admire or love, and who want the best for you, the next step is to attract their presence in your life. Let's start with a question: What do you think people care most about? Check only one response.

- ❏ My looks
- ❏ My intellect
- ❏ How much I care about them
- ❏ How much money I have

I believe the best answer is the third response. I like you if you make me like myself. The primary food that nurtures your relationships is your kindness. Joyful and kind attention and the practice of the five principles (gratitude, compassion, acceptance, meaning and forgiveness) help you express kindness. Life is simple when you keep these two thoughts: I go to work to practice kindness; I come home to practice kindness. When you align your day with the most pious intention, you practice kindness.

☺ Within relationships, three key ideas can help you offer kindness. See which one (or more) of the three you can practice today.

1. Truly see the goodness in others.
2. Remind others of their goodness.
3. Find others meaningful.

Next, we'll explore some ways you can include these ideas in your life.

> ✽ **Food for Thought:** I like you if you make me like myself.
> The primary food of your tribe is your kindness. ✽

Speak Kind Words

Your words have a life of their own. You inflict greater injury with your words than through your actions. An old teaching reminds me that the words

I choose should pass through three gates: They should be true, kind and necessary. Here are a few suggestions for choosing the kindest possible words amid disagreements.

Principle	Original version	More positive version
When talking about blame, phrase as a question rather than a fact.	"You don't know what you are doing."	"Do you think there is an easier way?"
Validate to the extent it is honest.	"What you are doing isn't working."	"You are doing it better than I could, but we probably need more help."
Try to understand.	"You shouldn't have been so rude to her."	"Did she upset you? You didn't seem too happy."
Use "I" language.	"You always make coffee colder and lighter than I like."	"I like my coffee hot and strong."

🖋 **Food for Thought:** The words I choose should pass through three gates: They should be true, kind and necessary. 🖋

In addition, try to use words that show your enthusiasm and gratitude rather than your burden. Here are two examples.

Original version	More positive version
I had to meet 12 clients today.	I was privileged to meet 12 clients today.
I have to meet my friend's parents.	I get to meet my friend's parents.

Now, on the next page, use these concepts to rewrite the following sentences.

Original version	My more positive version
I have to stay with my in-laws this weekend.	
I have to see my doctor next week.	
I have to take the kids to their activities every night this week.	
You are lazy.	
I don't like your cooking.	
Your snoring bothers me.	

Consider your words your gift to the world. Give kind gifts.

Listen More

You have two ears and one mouth. Listen at least twice as much as you speak. Your listening is likely to heal even more than the words you speak.

Listening is an active process. Help the speaker by showing your active engagement. Use attentive body language: nod, smile and make direct eye contact. Avoid distractions such as checking email or mail or looking at the TV or computer screen when you're listening to someone else.

Delay the urge to interrupt unless you have very good reason to do so. For a complex topic, summarize what you heard. An intelligent summary shows the speaker that you are engaged in the conversation. It will also ensure that you understand what is being said.

A common mistake is to try to solve a problem before you understand its full complexity. One way to prevent this is to have a clear line of communication. At the start of a meaningful conversation, consider asking something like, "Do you want me to just listen or try to solve the problem?" Most people will appreciate your candor and will let you know.

Ask appropriate questions. How interested and engaged you are in the conversation will come through in the quality of your questions. Everyone likes to be understood. People will be much more open to your opinion if they feel that theirs has been heard. Listen even if you have to speak. Your words sometimes are a gift; your listening always is.

> ✐ **Food for Thought:** Your words sometimes are a gift;
> your listening always is. ☞

☺ In your next conversation, practice a few of these ideas. Check the ones you agree with and add your own.

❏ Nod, smile and make eye contact.
❏ Minimize distractions (email, mail, TV).
❏ Avoid interrupting.
❏ Reflect back what I heard.
❏ Ask appropriate questions.
❏ Don't try to prematurely solve the problem.
❏ Understand before wanting to be understood.
❏ Assume good intent.
❏ Other ideas _____
❏ Other ideas _____
❏ Other ideas _____

Communicate

When you share, you invite others into your circle. You send a message that they are important to you, both for receiving your information and for providing valuable feedback. I have caused many more misunderstandings in my personal and professional life by *not* communicating than I have by communicating.

In terms of shared information, your relationship with a person has four boxes:

A. Information you both know	B. Information only the other person knows
C. Information only you know	D. Information you both don't know

(Note: This is a modification of the Johari Window model. Luft, Joseph. *Of Human Interaction*. New York, N.Y.: The McGraw-Hill Companies. © 1969. Used with permission.)

The bigger box A is, the healthier your relationship. Humans instinctively fill in the missing information with negative thoughts. That approach increases misunderstandings. Be proactive in sharing. Minimize the need for others to guess. ☺ Here are a few ideas to increase the size of box A. Write some facts in the second column that you think your loved one doesn't know about you and you feel comfortable sharing.

My dad	
My mom	
My ancestral home	
My quirks	

My dream job	
My high school fantasies	
My lucky number	
My secret wish	
My cravings	
What I enjoy doing most	
My favorite vacation spot	
Movies I love to watch	
Someone I secretly envy and why	
My most disappointing vacation	
Why I get out of bed each morning	

Praise

Let me share a secret about myself: I like those who make me like myself. I suppose that's true for you, too. We all enjoy a pat on the back for a job well-done, with one caveat: The praise has to be authentic. If someone praises you just because he or she wants something from you, then that praise will be annoying.

Here are a few ideas related to praise. Check the ones you agree with and add your own.

- ❑ Liberally praise the values a person stands for.
- ❑ Be discreet when admiring how attractive someone looks, particularly in a formal setting.
- ❑ Appreciate the effort, no matter the outcome.
- ❑ Mix your praise with gratitude.
- ❑ Make extra effort to praise people you think don't often receive praise.
- ❑ Praise a behavior you intend to encourage, particularly with children.
- ❑ Be authentic in your praise.
- ❑ Praise with no intention for personal gain.
- ❑ Praise to inspire not inflate.
- ❑ Other ideas _____
- ❑ Other ideas _____
- ❑ Other ideas _____

You can choose to see others' weaknesses as strengths or otherwise. Try to appreciate strengths as strengths. In addition, find how weaknesses can also be strengths. If someone has a Type A personality and always seems pressured to get things done, you may see this as a weakness. But maybe it's a strength: It might be how he or she accomplishes daily tasks. If your significant other is easygoing, maybe that's a perfect antidote to your perfectionist disposition. Two perfectionists who are busy trying to improve each other smells more of adrenaline than of the bonding hormone oxytocin.

On the next page, see how rephrasing a perceived weakness can help you see it in a positive light.

Judgmental words	Positive reframe
Rigid	Disciplined
Pushy	Confident
Careless	Carefree
Unsure	Flexible
Boring	Simple
Lazy	Easygoing
Greedy	Ambitious
Compulsive	Conscientious
Other ideas	Other ideas
Other ideas	Other ideas
Other ideas	Other ideas

☺ Pick someone new or familiar you'll meet today or in the next few days. Do your homework to learn the praiseworthy aspects of that person. It'll help you start and maintain the conversation and win more friends.

Laugh

Hearts that laugh together start beating together. Shared laughter and tears both create social bonding. Laughter is less about what's funny and more about connection, shared meaning, courtesy and feeling relaxed in another person's presence. An unexpected and sudden shift in perspective or an unrealistic exaggeration and relief can produce a giggle. Here are a few ways you can harness the value of humor in your community. Check the ones you agree with and add your own suggestions.

- ❏ Laugh with, not at.
- ❏ When unsure, direct a pun at yourself.
- ❏ Use care in humor: Use it in the right place, at the right time, in the right dose.
- ❏ Avoid practical jokes.
- ❏ Use humor to create social bonding.
- ❏ Place humor in the context of an ongoing dialogue.
- ❏ Don't let your jokes be a distraction from the main point.
- ❏ Be sensitive to the social context of the receiver.
- ❏ Be goofy at times.*
- ❏ Other ideas _____
- ❏ Other ideas _____
- ❏ Other ideas _____

*A few goofy actions I have (successfully) tried at home include wearing a silly hat, painting my face, walking around the house with a balloon tied to my eyeglasses, putting a sticky note on my forehead and putting a bowl on my head as a helmet.

Most of us aren't independently funny, but I believe that almost everyone can become better at sprinkling a little humor.

> 🕊 **Food for Thought:** Laughter is less about what's funny and more about connection, shared meaning, courtesy and feeling relaxed in another person's presence. 🕊

Be Flexible

Just as each petal of a flower is unique, every snowflake is distinct and every zebra has its signature stripes, we are all biologically different. Driven by our biology and upbringing, we all have unique preferences. Have you ever witnessed someone else's weird preferences, such as vacuuming twice a day even as an empty nester, driving 10 miles to save 2 cents on a gallon of gas or running on the treadmill at 2 a.m.? Do you have any unique preferences? Feel free to confess them in the box below.

My unique preferences

To the extent that you can, be flexible and accommodate other people's preferences by seeing them as different, not necessarily right or wrong.

☺ A perfect way to accommodate others' preferences is to remember small things. Most people are sensitive. When you remember others' preferences, such as the cereal they enjoy, the color they like or the aroma they love, they feel flattered by the attention. Your remembering small things like this says a lot. It shows you care; it makes others feel important. It'll also make you happier. Choose an important person in your life and try to gather his or her preferences in the space provided below and on the next page.

Name:	Relationship to me:
Favorite color	
Preferred fragrance	
How much he or she likes spices	

How much salt he or she likes on food	
Food cravings	
Books he or she likes to read	
Movie preferences or favorite actors	
Preferred room temperature	
How well he or she handles uncertainty	
Quirky habits or beliefs, such as sleeping facing the east or never yawning while eating	
Anything else	

If your spouse, partner or loved one were to give you 15 minutes of his or her time every day, what would you want? Rank in terms of your highest and lowest priorities.

Option	Rank
Spend quality time together at home.	
Get some long overdue work done.	
Go for a stroll.	
Shop online.	
Help with daily chores.	
Let my loved one do what he or she likes because it makes me happy to see him or her happy.	
Other	

Recognize that each of us has slightly different priorities and different strengths and expectations. If you can, try to satisfy your loved one's priorities at least a few days a week. Make an attempt to know what he or she prefers. Our instinct is to overdo what we feel capable of doing. This isn't a good investment of time. If you quench an unsatisfied desire in others, you will invite greater happiness in your life and strengthen your connections.

Find a Common Purpose

Shared purpose is the thread that stitches together the fabric of relationships. You are attracted to and find interesting the people with whom you have a shared purpose. Chance acquaintances become lasting relationships when you have common goals. Sharing a goal also takes away negative judgments. After an initial polite hello, shared purpose engages you in a longer, meaningful conversation.

Sometimes you may not be aware of this shared purpose right away. You may have to discover it by finding what's common between you and the other person. You can start with these 10 potential shared interests. Add more if you can.

Common hobbies	
Pets	
Common places we have visited overseas	
Similar books	

Common favorite foods	
A common social cause	
Kids of similar age	
Aligned work-related passions	
Birthplace	
Favorite sports team	
Other	
Other	
Other	
Other	

Finding shared experiences is a wonderful connector and can start a lifelong friendship.

Be Kind to Yourself

Kindness to the world starts with kindness to the self. Your relationships will weaken if you aren't kind to yourself. Ask yourself these two questions:

Am I doing something to myself that I would never do to someone else?	❑ Yes ❑ No
Am I letting someone else do something to me that I would never do to him or her?	❑ Yes ❑ No

If you answered yes to either of these, let's explore it further.

Am I doing something to myself that I would never do to someone else?
What is it?
Do I have a choice?
What choice(s) do I have?
What are the risks of the choice(s)?

Do I want to try the choice(s)?
If not, can I compensate myself in some other way?

Am I letting someone else do something to me that I would never do to him or her?

What is it?
Do I have a choice?
What choice(s) do I have?
What are the risks of the choice(s)?
Do I want to try the choice(s)?
If not, can I compensate myself in some other way?

Recognize that sometimes you have to put up with an indiscretion, at least for the short term. Keep your patience and try to dial down your sensitivity until you can mend the situation. One of my patients shared a wonderful metaphor that his grandma taught him: You can live your day wearing either a Velcro or a Teflon vest. The Velcro vest allows everything to stick to it, while the Teflon vest deflects everything. Try to wear the Teflon vest when you're surrounded by unreasonable, insensitive people.

☺ In the space provided below, make note of situations in which you will try to wear the Teflon vest.

I will wear the Teflon vest in these situations:

Each of these ideas originates in the five core principles: gratitude, compassion, acceptance, meaning and forgiveness. Living your life with these principles is the most important step you can take to seed and feed your relationships.

Despite your most well-meaning efforts, however, your garden will grow weeds that you will need to remove. These weeds can usurp your happiness if you don't remove them in time. This brings us to the next section of cultivating your tribe: keeping it relatively weed-free.

Weed

The Rules of Argument

Just as volcanoes prevent earthquakes, arguments serve a purpose. They allow you to release steam. Arguing is also better than punching someone in the nose! At the same time, explosive arguments aren't desirable.

☺ When you have no choice but to argue, try to use these rules to make your arguments more civil and productive. Add your thoughts about these rules in the third column below and the following two pages.

Rule	Perspective/example	My thought
Do not sacrifice a precious relationship for a material thing.	▶ Relationships take years to form but are just one argument away from breaking. ▶ The people in your life are your most precious asset.	
Understand before being understood.	▶ Most people like to be understood. ▶ Give others the gift of your understanding. ▶ Avoid practicing selective hearing. ▶ Do not jump to conclusions based on incomplete information.	
Stick to the point.	▶ Focus on the issue. ▶ Do not globalize an argument beyond the present point (for example, "You always say this"; "You never do this").	
Avoid e-arguments.	▶ Avoid arguing over email or by phone or text. Email and text are particularly bad because they can leave a permanent record. ▶ For minor issues, discussion in public may limit how loud anyone's voice can be.	

The Rules of Argument (continued)

Choose your words carefully.	▶ Use "I" language, rather than the accusatory "You" language (for example, "I feel hurt" versus "You hurt me"). ▶ Do not use words you will regret later.	
Keep the context in mind.	▶ Think about the context of the disagreement. ▶ Imagine what you would have done if you were in the other person's shoes. ▶ Validate. ▶ Validate even more.	
Limit your disagreement to the issue at hand.	▶ If you end up not finding common ground, limit the conversation to the present issue. ▶ Do not consider the other person entirely wrong if he or she sees one detail differently.	
Don't argue in front of children.	▶ Children feel threatened if you argue in front of them. ▶ When you are upset, children assume it's their fault. ▶ Violent arguments send the wrong message to children.	

The Rules of Argument (continued)

Redial your expectations.	▶ Recognize that everyone is entitled to opinions and preferences. ▶ Assume that everyone is busy. Do not expect others to participate in everything that's important to you.
Keep a strategy to prevent an explosion.	▶ Take a break if you are reaching an explosive point. ▶ Shout into a pillow instead of at the person. ▶ One approach to diffuse negative thoughts is "serene": **S**top negative thoughts. **E**xhale deeply for a few breaths. **R**edirect thoughts to gratitude or compassion. **E**valuate present stressor using gratitude or compassion. **NE**gotiate the issue with a fresh perspective.

The Rules of Anger

On a few occasions my angry outbursts have helped, but I regret the vast majority of my outbursts. Perhaps your experience is similar.

Anger (A) or frustrations are felt when there is a mismatch between expectation (E) and reality (R). The greater the mismatch, the greater the anger or frustration. The formula is: $A = E - R$. This simple formula leads to simple solutions.

You can change the reality (which often isn't in your control) or lower your expectations (which are often in your control).

Despite your efforts to optimize your expectations, you'll fall into the anger trap because your mind keeps increasing expectations as the world rises to meet them. Not all is lost in anger. In fact, you can harness the energy of your anger so that it helps and doesn't hurt as much. In the next exercise, try to use these rules for handling anger. Add your thoughts on each rule in the third column.

Rule	Perspective/example	My thought
Get angry with the right person.	▶ Do not substitute blame. ▶ Do not target someone just because he or she is weak or can't fight back. ▶ You can be judged better by how you treat the weak, not the strong.	
Get angry at the right place.	▶ Avoid spewing anger in public. ▶ Avoid getting angry in front of children or loved ones.	
Get angry at the right time.	▶ Do not show anger to someone who is already hurt or suffering. ▶ Do not show anger when someone is celebrating or on special days, such as a birthday or anniversary. ▶ Do not get angry when you don't have time to discuss the reason for your anger or its remedy.	

The Rules of Anger (continued)

Get angry to the right extent.	▶ Do not act with more anger than you feel. ▶ Do not react violently to a minor mistake.	
Get angry with the right intention.	▶ Do not use anger to simply hurt someone else. ▶ Do not use anger to vent your frustration. ▶ Direct your anger to inspire others and to help or correct a situation.	

If you follow these five rules, your anger will more likely serve a larger purpose. The next time you start to feel angry, run through this checklist.

Am I getting angry with the right person?	❏ Yes ❏ No
Is this the right place?	❏ Yes ❏ No
Is the time right for my anger?	❏ Yes ❏ No
Is my anger proportionate to the issue?	❏ Yes ❏ No
Do I have the right intention?	❏ Yes ❏ No

If you answer yes to all of the questions in this checklist, chances are that you won't regret your anger, and your anger, in the long term, will increase happiness.

The Rules of Critique

Critiques aren't pleasant to hear. The bitter pill of critique, however, needs to be given and swallowed. It helps if the pill is sugar coated, appropriately sized, gulped with plenty of water, and taken or given only when you must. If overdosed, this pill causes side effects. In the exercise that follows, try these ground rules for a healthy critique. Add your thoughts on each rule in the third column.

Rule	Perspective/example	My thought
Is it worth critiquing?	▶ Is the benefit worth the cost?	
Does the other person know more than I do?	▶ Consider that the other person's behavior may reflect that he or she knows more than you do.	
Does the other person know less than I do?	▶ Consider that the other person's behavior may reflect that he or she is unaware of a fact that you know.	

The Rules of Critique (continued)

Give others a fair hearing.	▶ Start with a question rather than a conclusion. ▶ Before you launch into your critique, allow the other person to explain his or her position.	
Reflect on the process rather than the person.	▶ When critiquing, focus on how the process went wrong rather than putting the blame on the person.	
Use the kindest words possible.	▶ Choose your words very carefully. ▶ Be kind in your expression.	
Do not critique someone who is already feeling bad about him- or herself.	▶ Your critique will hurt twice as much and provide half the benefit if you make it when someone is already feeling bad about him- or herself.	

The Rules of Critique (continued)

Limit your critique to one or two issues at most.	▶ Critique is tiring to hear. In one sitting, limit your critique to as few issues as possible. After your critique, check if it was helpful before discussing further.	
Be brief and to the point.	▶ A critique is less helpful when it becomes drawn out and padded. To avoid this, limit your critique to no more than a few minutes.	
Use your critique to inspire.	▶ Critiquing is an opportunity. ▶ Every critique should be directed to help others grow.	

If you're the person receiving a critique, remember these important points.

▶ Consider it a gift, to be used now or later. Accept it with grace.

▶ Focus more on what you can learn rather than on feeling hurt. Ask yourself, *What is the lesson here?* Don't discredit the person critiquing you.

▶ Remember that the person critiquing you would rather praise you. Critiquing someone is stressful.

- Try not to immediately counter each critique with an explanation. Be receptive and allow the other person to complete his or her thought.
- Finally, be willing to criticize your own actions. Laugh at yourself; if you don't, someone else surely will.

> 🕊 **Food for Thought:** Be willing to criticize your own actions. Laugh at yourself; if you don't, someone else surely will. 🕊

The Rules for Saying No

Saying no is a necessary evil. Although you need it to keep your life sane, the process of saying no isn't very pleasant. Your relationship becomes vulnerable when you say no, so use *no* gingerly. I really like the idea of a sandwiched *no*, which follows the sequence of yes-no-yes. The best way to understand this is through an example.

Situation: Your significant other calls you at work and wants to join you for lunch. But you would rather work through your lunch hour. What's the best way to say no so it doesn't hurt your loved one's feelings?

Option 1: Sorry, I can't come. I'm too busy.

Option 2: I would love to join you, but I'm really overcommitted right now. How about getting together for coffee at 4 p.m.?

You might say the first option is fine, and it might be, in a close relationship with plenty of understanding. But I believe the second option will be more useful in preventing your relationships from breaking. There are times when adding a few extra words can do wonders to avoid future misunderstandings.

Notice what I did with the second option: I surrounded the no with two yeses. I have tried this many times, and it works well. Let's practice these two scenarios.

Scenario 1: Your cousin wants you to join his family this Thanksgiving. You really like him but would rather spend time with your children at home. How do you respond? Use the space provided on the next page to write what you would say to your cousin.

Initial yes: Show your enthusiasm.	
Sandwiched no: Say that you can't come, perhaps with a reason.	
Final yes: Give an alternate option.	

Scenario 2: Your friend wants to invite your daughter for a sleepover. You trust and like your friend but aren't prepared to send your daughter to her house for a sleepover. How do you respond?

Initial yes: Show your enthusiasm.	
Sandwiched no: Say that you can't send your daughter for the sleepover, perhaps with a reason.	
Final yes: Give an alternate option.	

Try the sandwiched *no* next time you have to decline an offer. See if it works for you.

The Rules for Apology

No matter how hard you try to be perfect in everything, embody higher principles and live in the moment, you will mess up. I can guarantee this from personal experience. Your true test is how you handle your mistakes. A common error after making a mistake is to frantically search for an external reason for the mistake and transfer the blame as soon as possible. While it might save your ego for the short term, it won't help you grow. It also won't boost your self-esteem or self-control. This is the response of the weak. The strong respond by owning up to the mistake or at least to their own failing, apologizing for it and learning from it.

The next question is this: How should you apologize? You've probably guessed by now that I will offer some rules. Add your thoughts on each rule in the third column.

Rule	Perspective/example	My thought
Keep it short and simple.	▶ Don't beat around the bush. Be straightforward.	
An apology isn't an explanation.	▶ Keep explanations to a minimum when apologizing. Explanations show that you don't own your mistake.	
Do not counter-blame.	▶ An apology that ends with blaming the other person isn't an apology. ▶ An apology is just an apology. Period.	

The Rules of Apology (continued)

Pair your apology with something to make the situation better.	▶ A tangible action that goes beyond words shows that you're serious about your apology.	
Do something tangible to prevent repeating the mistake.	▶ Even more than your words, your actions will convince the other person that your apology is sincere.	

✍ **Food for Thought:** Your true test is how you handle your mistakes. ☜

Lower Your Expectations

Answer these questions about yourself.

Am I fairly busy on most days?	❑ Yes ❑ No
Do I have an hour to spare on most days?	❑ Yes ❑ No
Do I try to do the best I can?	❑ Yes ❑ No
Am I unable to get to some things despite my best intentions?	❑ Yes ❑ No
Do I always try to do the right thing?	❑ Yes ❑ No

Most people answer no to the second question and yes to the others. If this is true for you, it's likely true for everyone.

People are phenomenally busy. An average person has about 150 undone tasks at any point. Most people have a set of open files and black holes and are trying to protect their vulnerable selves.

Unrealistic expectations can lead to broken relationships. Low expectations give everyone room to breathe and prevent disappointments and anger. Keep measured expectations to increase the love you give and receive. That'll help you create stronger connections.

• • •

I wish you the very best in your efforts to seed, feed and weed your tribe.

TRY THIS TODAY

Call one of your friends or a loved one today and have a good heart-to-heart chat.

The Third Step:
Start a Mind-Body Practice

Week 9: Mind-Body Practices

A relaxed mind is a humble mind that isn't struggling with fear, greed or selfishness. Such a mind is happy. Many different paths converge to a similar state of the relaxed mind.

What Do You Do to Relax?

From the list below, pick the top five activities you do to relax.

- ❏ Read
- ❏ Exercise
- ❏ Music
- ❏ Art
- ❏ Prayer
- ❏ Meditation
- ❏ Yoga
- ❏ Muscle relaxation
- ❏ Tai chi
- ❏ Qi gong
- ❏ Relaxation tape
- ❏ Deep breathing
- ❏ Biofeedback
- ❏ Play with children
- ❏ Other _____
- ❏ Other _____
- ❏ Other _____
- ❏ Other _____

Each of these activities, when experienced nonjudgmentally, takes your brain into the focused mode. For an approach to work for you, it needs to fulfill three criteria. Check the criteria that apply to the activities you selected.

❏ You believe that the program will work for you.
❏ The philosophy of the program aligns with your worldview.
❏ You have the time and ability to practice this approach.

In the rest of this section, I will discuss a few practical aspects of meditation, one of the exercises on the list.

What Is Meditation?

Meditation is intentional relaxed presence with a compassionate, nonjudgmental and grateful disposition. This definition encompasses a plethora of states that range from the momentary calm someone experiences through a casual meditation practice to the ecstatic bliss an advanced yoga master experiences after a lifetime of training.

Meditation includes three different states that show progress in your practice.

1. **Sensory withdrawal.** There is a general disengagement from sensory input, including quieting of the mind's activity. You experience a state of calm that can last for minutes to hours after completing the practice.

2. **Sustained attention.** With freedom from the senses and its own wanderings, the mind achieves a single focus and keeps that focus for at least a few minutes, until it's interrupted by its wanderings or another sensory phenomenon. The relaxing effect may last the whole day.

3. **Immersion.** With training, you can effortlessly enter sustained attention within moments of starting the practice. Periodically, with a deep focus, you experience an ethereal lightness of the body with an intense awareness, total presence and a feeling of bliss. You can sustain this state anywhere from several minutes to hours. This state of immersion takes years of disciplined practice and moral living. The relaxing effect may last for days.

Types of Meditation

Meditation consists of four different practices. Individuals often combine these practices based on their preferences.

1. Attention-based meditation

In this practice, the primary focus is on training attention. You choose the object you use to train your attention. It could be related to faith or may simply be repeating the word *one*. Attention-based meditation is of two types:

Focused-attention meditation involves choosing to keep your focus for a certain amount of time. You may focus on something external, such as an image or sound, or internal, such as your breath, a word or a sentence. The focused attention, although intentional, is relaxed.

Open-monitoring meditation is nonjudgmental awareness of sensory input and thoughts at each moment. It is a state of nonreactive awareness to the contents of your conscious experience, whatever they are. Your meditation may evolve to open monitoring after years of focused-attention practice.

2. Feeling-based meditation

In this practice, your primary focus is on cultivating a desirable feeling, such as loving kindness, gratitude or compassion. Attention training is a secondary component, although it happens on its own in the background. You may focus on a particular individual who is suffering, carrying the intention to decrease the suffering, or focus on the world at large.

3. Thought-based meditation

In this introspective meditation style, you choose a thought and think about it, excluding every other thought. The intention is to reach a deep insight into the thought and, through that process, into the nature of reality. The selected thought generally is inspirational in nature and not purposeless mind wandering. The process naturally trains attention and helps cultivate wisdom.

4. Meditation as a Background Practice

Several relaxing mind-body approaches use meditation as a background practice. These include tai chi, qi gong, guided imagery, progressive muscle relaxation, and even music and artwork. I regard these as mild states of meditation. Joyful and kind attention also can be included in this group of practices.

Meditation: The First Step

The primary requirement and goal of meditation is a calm, focused, relaxed mind. But how can you cultivate a calm, focused, relaxed mind? A familiar metaphor may help.

Think of your mind as a lake. The calm surface of the lake is disturbed when you throw pebbles in it. These pebbles are fear, greed and selfishness. You can avoid some of the pebbles, but you can't wish them all away. One way to help your mind is by cultivating greater equanimity.

Equanimity doesn't mean you don't care. Instead, it's an inner flexibility in your preferences. It recognizes that just as you didn't control which set of chromosomes collaborated one remarkable day to create you, you can't control how long your life will be and, to some extent, the path your life will take. Equanimity helps you love most intensely; and when the time comes, it helps you say goodbye, until we meet again. Equanimity stops your struggle with what is.

A lack of equanimity can lead to excessive self-focus, lack of contentment and many negative emotions, particularly fear. Fear that protects you from a real threat is helpful. But fear that saps your energy and promotes inaction hurts you in many ways. This is what makes equanimity desirable.

I believe equanimity has two paths: wisdom and love. The path of wisdom has each of the principles (gratitude, compassion, acceptance, meaning and forgiveness) as its key milestones. It progresses to a point where you get total clarity for the three questions related to meaning: *Who am I? Why am I here?* and *What is this world?* This wisdom overcomes fear.

The other path is of love that transforms itself into surrender. Surrender to what? To a reality higher than our minds. But surrendering to a higher reality isn't easy, because you can't experience this reality with the five senses. For love to transform into surrender, it needs to be infused with gratitude, acceptance and selflessness, all of which are planned by the power to which you offer your surrender: grace.

Meditation Programs

Meditation has as many styles as there are people who meditate. Every person has a unique approach. Here I will share with you a few breath-based meditation programs I have personally practiced and found helpful for myself and others.

I consider deep breathing as the anchor of most meditation practices. It can also be your primary personal practice. Natural breathing serves a biological purpose. Breathing that's intentional and refined into deep, relaxing breaths can also serve an emotional and spiritual purpose.

Common to all breath-based meditation programs is a suggestion to breathe diaphragmatically. One good way to practice diaphragmatic breathing is to imagine filling a cup with water when you inhale. Just as you fill a cup from the bottom up, fill your lower lungs and then your upper lungs. First expand your belly by moving your diaphragm and then your chest. You can keep your hands on your belly and pay attention to your belly's movement when you inhale. When you exhale, just as the cup empties from top down, empty your upper lungs first and then your lower lungs. If any of this seems confusing, just take deep and slow breaths in a way that feels comfortable to you.

The first exercise will help you observe your breath at the tip of your nose.

☺ **Exercise 1: Breath Awareness A**

1. Sit in a comfortable, dimly lit, quiet and safe place with your eyes closed. You can choose any posture you like other than lying on the bed. Avoid doing this exercise immediately after a heavy meal.

2. Spend the first two minutes paying attention to all of the sounds you hear in the environment. Allow your awareness to travel to the source of the sounds. Try to avoid making any judgments about the sounds.

3. At this point, gradually settle your awareness and bring it to your breath.

4. Practice deep, slow, diaphragmatic breathing for the rest of the exercise.

5. Breathe at a rate and depth that feels comfortable.

6. Visualize your breath at the tip of your nostrils. Feel the subtle, cool breath as it flows in and a warm, cozy breath as you breathe out.

7. Keep your attention at the tip of the nostrils for the next few minutes, visualizing the inward- and outward-flowing breath.

8. Now allow your breath to become increasingly subtle until you just about stop feeling the flow.

9. Keep your awareness on the tip of the nostrils with this subtle breath for the next few minutes.

10. Continue this exercise for as long as you like, at least 10 minutes.

In the next exercise, we'll track the movement of the breath.

☺ Exercise 2: Breath Awareness B

1. Sit in a comfortable, dimly lit, quiet and safe place with your eyes closed. You can choose any posture you like, other than lying on the bed. Avoid doing this exercise immediately after a heavy meal.

2. Spend the first two minutes paying attention to all of the sounds you hear in the environment. Allow your awareness to travel to the source of the sounds. Try to avoid making any judgments about the sounds.

3. At this point, gradually settle your awareness and bring it to your breath.

4. Practice deep, slow, diaphragmatic breathing for the rest of the exercise.

5. Breathe at a rate and depth that feels comfortable.

6. Visualize your inhaled breath traveling from the tip of your nose to the farthest reaches of your upper body (head, neck and chest).

7. Now visualize your exhaled breath traveling from your upper body out to the tip of the nose.

8. Visualize your inhaled breath traveling from the tip of your nose to the farthest reaches of your lower body (belly and legs).

9. Now visualize your exhaled breath traveling from your lower body out and up to the tip of the nose.

10. Repeat this exercise for as long as you like, at least for 10 minutes.

These breathing exercises have many variants, so change and adapt them as you like. If you wish to learn more-advanced techniques, it may help to work with a trained teacher. One simple variation is to pay attention to the movements of your abdomen instead of the tip of the nose. Another common approach is to pay attention to the pause between when you inhale and when you exhale, and deliberately increase that pause within your range of comfort.

In the next exercise, focus on body awareness. Your body offers an excellent focus for attention that's always available and enjoys the relaxation that comes with paying attention.

☺ **Exercise 3: Body Awareness in Five Breaths**
1. Sit in a comfortable, dimly lit, quiet and safe place with your eyes closed. You can choose any posture you like, other than lying on the bed. Avoid doing this exercise immediately after a heavy meal.

2. Spend the first two minutes paying attention to all of the sounds you hear in the environment. Allow your awareness to travel to the source of the sounds. Try to avoid making any judgments about the sounds.

3. At this point, gradually settle your awareness and bring it to your breath.

4. Practice deep, slow, diaphragmatic breathing for the rest of the exercise.

5. Breathe at a rate and depth that feels comfortable.

6. Take a deep breath as you bring your awareness to your head. Imagine your brain filling up with soothing white light. Gradually exhale this breath.

7. Take a deep breath as you bring your awareness to your face and neck. Imagine your face and neck filling up with soothing white light. Gradually exhale this breath.

8. Take a deep breath as you bring your awareness to your chest. Imagine your chest filling up with soothing white light. Gradually exhale this breath.

9. Take a deep breath as you bring your awareness to your belly. Imagine your belly filling up with soothing white light. Gradually exhale this breath.

10. Take a deep breath as you bring your awareness to your entire body. Imagine your entire body filling up with soothing white light. Gradually exhale this breath.

11. Continue this exercise for as long as you like. Aim for 10 sets, which will take about 10 minutes.

A common variation of this exercise is to focus only on one part of your body and try to relax it instead of practicing deep breathing at the same time. I prefer to combine body visualization and deep breathing.

Breath and body exercises have countless variations. A paced breathing meditation program called Mayo Clinic Meditation is available on a DVD and also as a smartphone app. This program takes you through three minutes of paced breathing and one minute of silent meditation in three cycles. The total practice is 15 minutes.

In any practice, the key principles are to keep the exercises simple, do enough repetitions and persevere. Choose only a few exercises for daily practice to help keep your time commitment realistic. As you learn and experience these exercises, keep your primary goal clear: to cultivate a deeper, kinder attention. With this attention, extraneous thoughts will fade. As you progress along this path, you'll become your own teacher and find new ways to refine your attention.

Each of the five principles also lends itself to meditation practice. For example, here is one related to compassion.

☺   **Exercise 4: Compassion Meditation**
1. Sit in a quiet, safe place with your eyes closed.
2. Settle into slow, deep breathing for a few minutes.
3. Draw an imaginary circle.
4. Place yourself in that circle.
5. Within that circle also include someone you dearly love.
6. Create positive warm feelings for that person.
7. Now focus on how the two of you are similar. You're both humans. You have similar biologic needs (food, breath, healthy body). You both need security, care and love. Do you have similar preferences for food? Do you both like to travel? Do you like similar clothes? Are your movie choices similar? Try to find similarities even in differences. Do you both have unique idiosyncrasies? Are you both similar in having dissimilar preferences?
8. Now with each breath you take in, imagine you're bringing that person love and healing from the world. Each time you breathe out, imagine taking away that person's pain and suffering.
9. Continue slow, deep breathing throughout this exercise.

Helpful Tips

Whether you are just starting your meditation practice or are an experienced practitioner, you'll experience several challenges throughout your meditation career. Physical fatigue and most other uncontrolled symptoms (such as severe pain, shortness of breath, nausea and itching) interfere with meditation practice. Physical comfort will help enhance your focus.

You might move back and forth between laziness one day and too much enthusiasm the next. Both can damage your meditation practice. Calm alertness is the ideal state of the mind.

If you expect to achieve an immersive experience with a profound sense of bliss within a week of starting meditation, you will be disappointed. Undoing your mind's lifelong tendency toward mental time travel takes years to overcome. Achieving a brief period of calm and clarity is a reasonable short-term goal. Try not to win the meditation Olympics. In meditation, the ones who let go of winning as a goal are the ones who win.

> 🕊 **Food for Thought:** Undoing your mind's lifelong tendency toward mental time travel takes years to overcome. Achieving a brief period of calm and clarity is a reasonable short-term goal. 🕊

Deep breathing and relaxation will invariably put you to sleep. In almost every group meditation practice, I hear the sweet sound of someone's snores. It only shows that people have a sleep debt to pay. With time, you'll be able to stay awake, yet calm and relaxed.

The mind's innate restlessness pulls you into all kinds of stories. The mind loves to weave stories when you sit in meditation. You'll have to be patient with your mind. Observe its activity. Smile. Gently re-engage with your practice. Your mind will gradually yield. I have provided some additional tips below to help influence your mind.

Ego, particularly your spiritual ego, will be your final challenge as you advance in your practice. With progress, you risk considering yourself better than others. This is a sure way to stifle further growth. You have to balance your self-confidence with humility. The company of a well-meaning teacher or friend who has tread this path can do wonders to help you stay aligned.

Here are a few additional suggestions with the rationale that supports them.

Suggestion	Rationale
Keep yourself physically fit.	Meditation often is practiced in a sitting posture, preferably with your back straight. Physical fitness will help. Early in your practice, support your back against a wall or the back of a chair.

Suggestion *(cont.)*	Rationale *(cont.)*
Practice in a safe, quiet place.	This will decrease your need to monitor the world for safety and will also limit your sensory load.
Start with 15 minutes a day.	Avoid an hourlong meditation practice in the first month. Start with 15 minutes a day and build gradually.
Be consistent.	A regular time, place and practice will help you cultivate discipline.
Balance your life.	Simplify your life, but not to the point of depriving yourself of basic necessities (and some luxuries).
Start by remembering someone you admire.	Thinking about someone you truly respect will focus your practice and decrease your mind's distractions.
Assign meaning to your practice.	Dedicating the benefits of your practice to a cause higher than yourself, such as the well-being of children, will help you remain focused and disciplined.
Maintain a log of your distracting thoughts.	Keep a diary with you to write, particularly if a distracting thought keeps plaguing your mind.
Combine meditation with prayer.	Deepen your practice by aligning your faith with your meditation practice; do this by choosing an appropriate image or sound.

One final thought: Make others around you comfortable with your practice, particularly those who don't know much about meditation or might have some misconceptions about it. Let them know that you're not leaving the material world, changing your clothes to a saffron robe or embracing a New Age practice to have mystical experiences. Meditation has now been tested in many research studies and is considered scientific- and evidence-based.

From here, you may ask yourself, *How do I know if meditation is working for me?*

How to Know If Meditation Is Working for You

The most important goal of meditation is to become kinder — to yourself and to others. If meditation isn't making you kinder, then it isn't working for you. To the best of your ability, answer the questions below and on the next page after a few months of practice. Ask your friends and loved ones for help when needed.

Am I becoming calmer?	❑ Yes ❑ No
Am I more flexible now?	❑ Yes ❑ No
Do I feel happier?	❑ Yes ❑ No
Am I becoming more forgiving?	❑ Yes ❑ No
Am I less forgetful?	❑ Yes ❑ No
Am I noticing more things?	❑ Yes ❑ No
Do I feel physically healthier?	❑ Yes ❑ No
Do I have more energy at the end of the day?	❑ Yes ❑ No
Am I less bothered by daily annoyances?	❑ Yes ❑ No
Do I look forward to each day?	❑ Yes ❑ No
Do I look forward to meditating?	❑ Yes ❑ No
Is my sleep more restful?	❑ Yes ❑ No
Do I feel more spiritual?	❑ Yes ❑ No
Do I feel more in control of my thoughts?	❑ Yes ❑ No

Is my thinking becoming clearer?	❏ Yes ❏ No
Am I more creative?	❏ Yes ❏ No
Do I find myself thinking about meditation?	❏ Yes ❏ No
Have I suggested meditation to someone?	❏ Yes ❏ No

All of these have been my personal experiences and the experiences of those who have shared their progress with me. Not everyone will attain all of these benefits. Be patient. Most important, be kind to yourself and do not postpone happiness. That's where it all starts, doesn't it?

I hope you enjoy your personal meditation practice.

TRY THIS TODAY

Make time for a meditation break. If you already meditate regularly, try some of the approaches discussed in this section to deepen your practice.

The Fourth Step:
Pick Healthy Habits

Week 10: Healthier You—Take Small Steps

In this final section, I would like to share some healthy habits and fun ideas that may help you decrease your stress and increase the energy available to you each day. These are broad suggestions, so feel free to modify them based on your life situation.

Read Good Books

Books are low-cost, low-tech tools that can connect you with some of the best minds of the world at your leisure and in your home. Reading a good book is a perfect attention-training exercise.

☺ Make a list of the books you would love to read. Ask like-minded people for ideas; visit the local library and search for different genres and fields, not just the types of books you're used to reading. Join a book club to instill discipline. If you can't find a book club, start your own.

List of the books I want to read this year	
Title	**Author**

List of the books I want to read this year (continued)	
Title	**Author**

Once you befriend books, you won't ever feel lonely for the rest of your life.

Do a Few Things You've Always Wanted to Do

Many of us carry a secret wish list in our heads, but the items on the list get pushed down by the details of daily living.

☺ List the places you want to visit, people you want to meet and things you want to do by the end of your life. Let's start here. Check the things you plan to do in the next two years.

I definitely want to visit these places in my life:		❏
		❏
		❏
		❏
I definitely want to meet these people in my life:		❏
		❏
		❏
		❏

I definitely want to do these things in my life:		❏
		❏
		❏
		❏

Creating and using this list will enrich your life, make your years more memorable and give you a greater sense of fulfillment.

Decrease Your Dose of Daily News

A physician colleague who was trying to lose weight grumbled to me that he had no time to exercise. We sat down and found that on an average day, he was spending two hours watching news and eating mindlessly during that time. He was shocked by the revelation; he had no idea how he had gotten into this habit. He didn't even like it. By shedding this habit, he was able to add two hours to his day, much to the pleasure of his family.

How much time do you spend watching news?

	In the morning	During the day	At night
Amount of time (minutes)			

If the total time for each day adds up to more than 15 minutes, you can make some changes. For example, it's OK to check the news once or twice a day, but you don't have to check news headlines every 30 minutes. Exposure to too much negative news can disturb your sleep and hurt your health. Try to break that habit today before it takes any more time away from your family or self-care.

Take Care of Yourself

Speaking of self-care, do you take good care of your body and mind? Try to answer the questions on the next page.

Do I get at least seven to eight hours of restful sleep at night?	❏ Yes ❏ No
Am I able to exercise on most days of the week?	❏ Yes ❏ No
Have I been screened for preventable cancers?	❏ Yes ❏ No
Do I know my cholesterol, blood pressure and blood sugar levels?	❏ Yes ❏ No
Do I have any addictions (alcohol, tobacco or other substances)?	❏ Yes ❏ No
Have I taken a fun vacation in the last two years?	❏ Yes ❏ No
Have I spent time on an educational retreat?	❏ Yes ❏ No
Do I always wear a seat belt?	❏ Yes ❏ No
Do I drive within the speed limit?	❏ Yes ❏ No
Do I exercise self-control in my diet?	❏ Yes ❏ No
Do I laugh at least once on most days?	❏ Yes ❏ No
Do I relax my mind for at least 15 minutes on most days?	❏ Yes ❏ No
Do I have at least two people in my life I can trust?	❏ Yes ❏ No
Have I addressed my fears?	❏ Yes ❏ No
Do I belong to a group that helps me fulfill a higher meaning?	❏ Yes ❏ No

For each no you checked on this list, think about how you can address it in the next three months.

Decrease Your Screen Time

Whenever possible, try to experience the world in its full dimensions, not just the two dimensions of the screen. We spend more time watching screens than doing any other activity. Some screen time is necessary because it's part of our work, it's a way to communicate and it helps run our lives. My suggestion is to be more intentional about this time and decrease its dose if you can.

Check the options that sound good to you.		
Can I reduce my screen time? ❏ Yes ❏ No	Decrease unnecessary TV time.	❏
	Decrease the time I spend surfing the Internet at work and at home.	❏
	Stop checking email during every empty moment.	❏
	Don't look at the computer while talking on the phone with family and friends.	❏
	Other	❏
	Other	❏
	Other	❏
Can I add nonscreen time to my day? ❏ Yes ❏ No	Take a 10-minute stroll during my lunch hour.	❏
	Take a five-minute walking break every two to three hours.	❏
	Talk to someone I feel close to every day.	❏
	Always have an unfinished book nearby.	❏
	Other	❏
	Other	❏
	Other	❏
	Other	❏

The primary obstacle to decreasing screen time is feeling bored. We have come to hate getting bored. We try to fill every empty moment with a productive activity.

Allow yourself to be bored. Add empty time to your day's menu. Don't schedule any planning or problem-solving during this time. Just be. Practice joyful attention, appreciate the little wonders of the world — man-made or natural — with all your senses. Who knows what insight about team building a little colony of ants in your backyard may provide you.

Simplify Your Life
Avoid taking a bite bigger than you can swallow. As we climb the success ladder, luxuries become decencies, and decencies become necessities. In 1970, 3 percent of people viewed having a second television as a necessity. That number rose to 45 percent in 2000. The more stuff you have, the more time and energy you invest in maintaining it. If you need an extra 1,000 square feet of storage for possessions that you might need some day, it's time to take a good look at your life. Ask yourself, *Do I really need all this stuff?* If you haven't used a box of old clothing since your last move six years ago, it's unlikely you'll need it anytime soon (or in this lifetime).

A second and equally important aspect of simplification relates to your emotional life. Behaviors not accepted, people not forgiven, envies not overcome — our minds carry a long list of loads. Try to lighten your emotional load as much as you can. If you can't shed a load, try to at least shove it into your attic for now — if possible, for the next hour or for this day. Taking 15 minutes to just worry and solve problems so that you don't have to worry the rest of the day might help. I call this scheduled worry time.

Delegating your work, particularly aspects that are less critical, is an excellent way to take a load off your mind. When delegating, you'll have to let go of some control. You'll also have to accept that the same task can be done in different ways. The best managers are those who delegate so effectively that their absence is hardly felt.

Consider ways you can simplify your life with the exercise on the next page.

Check the options that appeal to you		
Can I simplify my material life? ❑ Yes ❑ No	Give away some of my stuff.	❑
	Put off getting more things for now.	❑
	Put limits on getting some of the things I want.	❑
	Delegate some of my work.	❑
	Other	❑
	Other	❑
	Other	❑
	Other	❑
Can I simplify my emotional life? ❑ Yes ❑ No	Live one day of the week in total forgiveness (Friday).	❑
	Live one day of the week in total acceptance (Wednesday).	❑
	Lower expectations of others.	❑
	Recognize and accept that I am imperfect.	❑
	Other	❑
	Other	❑
	Other	❑
	Other	❑

A simple life is one lived with humility, in balance with nature. It helps free up your time to pursue higher meaning. One helpful step to simplify your life is to choose only the battles worthy of your time.

Pick Your Battles

Identify your challenges and categorize them into one of the four quadrants.

	Controllable	Not as controllable
Important	A	B
Not as important	C	D

I have noted a few suggestions in the table below. You may or may not agree with all of them. Feel free to draw this table on a piece of paper and categorize your own challenges in the four boxes.

	Controllable	**Not as controllable**
Important	▶ Health ▶ Relationships ▶ Finances ▶ Work (a few issues) ▶ Spiritual growth	▶ The entire past ▶ Geopolitical issues ▶ Global warming ▶ Economy ▶ Taxes ▶ Others' behavior ▶ Traffic ▶ Weather ▶ Someone bad-mouthing me
Not as important*	▶ My teenager's hair color ▶ Friends coming late to my party ▶ My partner's choice of movies	▶ What others order at a restaurant ▶ A co-worker slurping coffee ▶ A co-worker's accent

*Note that I said,"Not as important," not "Not important."

This exercise is particularly helpful if you have a lot going on in your life, which may be a rule rather than an exception. The greatest stress comes from feeling overwhelmed by the present — we have too many balls up in the air. Letting a few (less important) balls drop may be essential to keeping the most important ones aloft. Choosing not to improve can be a great improvement. On the next page, you'll find a few suggestions to handle each of the quadrants.

	Controllable	**Not as controllable**
Important	▶ Take care of these aspects. ▶ Recognize that change often takes more time than desired.	▶ Learn from these. ▶ Bring acceptance and forgiveness.
Not as important*	▶ Consider cost vs. benefit. ▶ How meaningful is it? ▶ Let it go if the cost is greater than the benefit and it's not very meaningful.	▶ Let it go.

*Note that I said, "Not as important," not "Not important."

You have only a limited amount of physical, mental, emotional and spiritual energy. Apply your energy to the most significant problems that you can solve. Choose only those challenges that are worthy of your time based on their relevance and your ability to have an impact on them.

Lighten Up

We often take life more seriously than we need to. Humor brings you into intentional presence. Find ways to insert humor in your life. When adding humor, make sure your pun doesn't cross the line of decency and isn't directed at someone. Here are a few ideas to lighten up. Check the ones you think could help and add a few ideas of your own.

❑ Watch funny movies.
❑ Read humorous books.
❑ Watch funny TV shows.
❑ Laugh at yourself.
❑ Befriend lighthearted people.
❑ Find humor in children's innocent words.
❑ Other _____
❑ Other _____
❑ Other _____

You laugh more when you laugh together. Humor connects us with others. A good laugh can do wonders to ward off your fatigue, physical or emotional, and improves your relationships.

Be Prepared for an Amygdala Hijack

In order to survive, we had to excel at recognizing threats. Our brain is thus always alert for potential threats, including the threats of rejection and insults. The lower limbic brain scans the sensory input like a security system that's permanently turned on. This system is also very sensitive. The tiniest whiff of rejection is enough to excite it.

For this reason, no matter how much effort you put into cultivating patience and living your life immersed in the higher principles, you will fail. You will get angry, disappointed, worried and frustrated. That just goes with living in an imperfect world. When you're seething with anger or buried in worry, your amygdala — your fear center — hijacks the rest of the brain. In this state, the soup of chemicals that are released effectively paralyze the higher cortical part of the brain. Rationality is left far behind. Many unkind and irrational acts happen in this state and are often a source of later regret.

Plan ahead for these situations. Think back to the "serene" approach from Week 8 (page 189). Here is another version of the same approach, which is based on three key understandings:

1. When your rage is out of control, it's best to excuse yourself and take a break. While this may seem awkward, excusing yourself is better than showing your worst manners.
2. Your brain stops rational thinking when it is marinating in adrenaline soup. Deep breathing is the simplest and most effective way to dampen an adrenaline surge.
3. Thoughts of compassion can calm the angriest minds. Compassion shifts your attention away from personal frustration to the other person's challenges with an intention and effort to help.

To help remember this, I use what I call the ABCC approach.

Steps	Examples
1. **A**sk for a quick break	Ask for a bathroom break, take a walk, drink a glass of water, or ask to meet at a different time.
2. **B**reathe	Practice slow deep breaths for a few minutes.
3. **C**ompassion	Bring a compassionate thought for the person involved in the situation, or for someone else you know is suffering. Can you think of the children who will sleep hungry tonight, or the 4,500 people who will receive a new diagnosis of cancer today?
4. **C**ontext	Now with a clearer head, reframe the situation in a broader context. Can you see that the other person doesn't mean to hurt you but, instead, is trying to protect himself? Can you see an insulting expression as a call for help? Can you find meaning in the adversity? Can you feel grateful for all that is not wrong?

Re-engage with the situation once you have cooled down with the ABCC approach and can take a more mature look at the situation.

Eat a Healthy Diet

Physically and to some extent, emotionally, you become what you eat. That makes your diet extremely important. Three aspects to pay attention to are what you eat, how much you eat and how you eat.

What you eat. Eat a balanced diet. Choose whole grains, nuts, fish, vegetables, protein and fiber. Eat a variety of foods to get a broad range of nutrients. Avoid refined sugars, saturated fat, megadose vitamins and calorie-dense food. Eliminate trans fat.

How much you eat. How full you feel when you eat can be an inaccurate signal of how much you've eaten. This is especially true if you eat quickly and consume calorie-dense food. Fill only about 80 percent of your stomach. Stop eating when you feel just a little full. If you pause a few minutes after feeling lightly full, you will soon feel comfortably full. If you continue eating past that point, you'll feel stuffed pretty quickly.

How you eat. Like a Tyrannosaurus rex, we tend to eat big chunks of food, graze all day as cattle do and swallow food like the alligators do. We take in calories without even enjoying what we're eating. Such mindless eating leads to taking in too many calories. Instead, consider what I like to call a "slow-small-savor" approach. Eat *slowly*, chewing your food well. Take *small* bites. And *savor* each morsel. The slow-small-savor approach may help you get more out of your food and help you lose weight, too, if that's your goal.

In this exercise, be honest and commit to one change you can make in the next week.

	Areas for improvement	What I can improve in 1 week
What I eat		
How much I eat		
How I eat		

Your dinner plate is a work of magic; it's a joint effort of millions of men and women and elements of nature. Do it full justice by savoring each bite.

Keep Your Body Agile

Comfort and convenience lead to laziness and deconditioning. Remote controls, drive-thru everything, automobiles, elevators, too much screen time — all of these contribute to the fact that more than 80 percent of us currently do not get enough physical activity.

Each week, most healthy adults should get at least 150 minutes of moderate or 75 minutes of vigorous aerobic activity, in addition to muscle-strengthening exercises. If you need to, break your physical activity into small chunks and spread it throughout the day. Combine it with joyful attention. Take a walk in nature, park your car farther away from the store, walk up the stairs, walk to your co-worker's office instead of calling, schedule a meeting away from your office, walk to where you choose to eat, walk while talking on the phone in your office or at home, take a kind-attention stroll during the day, schedule a walking meeting, or join an athletic club — these are just some ideas to get you started.

Physical activity has many benefits. Almost everything that you want in life will be easier to achieve if you're more physically active. I encourage you to search online for the benefits and recommendations of physical activity beyond what you already know and then complete this exercise.

What are the benefits of increased physical activity?	
Am I meeting my physical activity goal?	
What can I do next week to increase my physical activity?	
How can I make physical activity more interesting?	

Get Enough Good-Quality Sleep

To be awake is human; to sleep is divine! We sleep on average one hour less than we did 20 years ago. Currently, more than half of us don't get enough sleep. Our sleep is also not restful. As a result, 1 in 4 of us feels drowsy during the day. This is more often related to lifestyle choices than to a sleep disorder. No wonder we consume more than 4 kilograms of coffee powder per person every year, and nearly 9 million Americans take prescription sleeping pills to help them sleep.

Sleep is brain food. Your brain and body age faster with lack of sleep. Not getting enough sleep can lead to weight gain, fatigue, loss of creativity, high blood pressure, diabetes, heart attack, stroke and accidents. Long-term lack of sleep can even be fatal.

Make sleep a priority. Consider it a sacred time. Maybe you already have a good sleeping schedule. If you don't, here are a few ideas that might help. Check which ones might work in your life and add a few ideas of your own.

- ❏ Avoid heavy meals or alcohol near bedtime.
- ❏ Avoid caffeine within four to six hours of bedtime.
- ❏ Exercise regularly, but avoid strenuous exercise within two hours of bedtime.
- ❏ Create a comfortable sleeping environment that's quiet, is the right temperature and has a comfortable bed.
- ❏ Try not to use your bedroom for office work or watching TV.
- ❏ If you can, try not to take your worries to bed with you.
- ❏ Relax your body and mind before going to sleep. A relaxing before-bedtime routine may include a warm bath, soothing reading, deep breathing or eating a light snack.
- ❏ If you can, try to decrease your need to wake up because of pain, a full bladder or heartburn.
- ❏ If a worry keeps bothering you, write it in a journal or try your best to postpone thinking about it until the morning.
- ❏ Do not go to bed hungry.
- ❏ Other _____
- ❏ Other _____

Everything you've learned in this book will take time and effort to bring into your life on a regular basis. Experts say it takes 10,000 hours of practice to master a skill. Some say it takes at least six months of effort to change a behavior. A key aspect to make and sustain a change is to develop a disciplined practice. The human mind resists attempts to change the status quo. A few props mentioned in this table may help. Choose the ones you can apply in your life and think of one or two more.

Prop	Rationale	
Work with a buddy.	▶ Make yourself externally accountable by partnering with someone who can cheer you on. ▶ A buddy also multiplies the ideas and helps when the going gets tough.	❑
Insert cues.	▶ Cues remind you to change a behavior. ▶ Cues start the chain for a new habit. ▶ The right cue will facilitate the behavior change.	❑
Use a daily journal.	▶ A journal can be your surrogate buddy. ▶ Journaling helps you log your progress. ▶ A journal can provide you with daily structure.	❑
Use rewards.	▶ Predictable rewards when you achieve certain milestones can motivate you. ▶ Plan a few surprise rewards.	❑
Other		❑
Other		❑

Discipline leads to intentionality. In terms of practice, the two words I use to describe the Resilient Living Program are *conscious living*. Conscious living means to become intentional about your thoughts and actions. It is living in harmony with nature and each other. When you choose consciously, you free yourself from short-term, comfort-seeking, unhealthy habits. That is your first step toward transformation.

I believe that by choosing some of the ideals of the Resilient Living Program, you have taken the first step toward experiencing sustained happiness. What's the second step? How about joining us?

🕊 **Food for Thought:** Conscious living means to become intentional about your thoughts and actions. 🖎

TRY THIS TODAY

In your mind or on paper, rank the healthy habits in order of the ones you do well to the ones that need the most improvement. Choose one healthy habit and think of ways you can make it a more regular part of your life.

Join Us

My colleagues and I strive to live each day of our lives according to the principles you've learned in this workbook. We hope to transform at least a small part of the world with principles-based living. I invite you to join us in our campaign to decrease global stress and anxiety and enhance the world's happiness, resilience and well-being. Here are a few steps you can take.

Educate yourself. Visit our interactive website at *www.stressfree.org*, our central place for archiving information, presenting data from our research studies, sharing announcements and offering online training.

Attend in-person workshops. We offer individual and group workshops across the United States and worldwide. The courses currently available are the Stress Management and Resiliency Training (SMART) program, the Transform course and online programs, including a 12-module Resilient Living course with videos, quizzes and practice exercises, shorter programs, quotes, blogs, tweets and other relevant material. Let us know if you are interested in any of these programs by visiting *www.stressfree.org/programs*.

Connect on Twitter. Follow me at @amitsoodmd.

Become a teacher. Contact us to learn how you can teach our program to others.

• • •

Whatever path you take, accept my invitation to immerse yourself in higher principles. I promise that the journey will be worth every bit of your effort. Start that journey today. Don't wait for the perfect sunny morning. Do not postpone joy; life is too short.

I feel privileged to greet you on this journey. Welcome! I wish you a lifetime of peace and happiness. The best way to not postpone joy is to make a commitment to kindness — toward others and toward yourself.

Appendix: Additional Attention Exercises

This appendix describes additional attention-training exercises. Try these exercises, identify the ones you find most appealing, and incorporate them into your daily schedule.

☺ Exercise 1. Find Uniqueness Within the Ordinary

Pick four similar-looking oranges (or any other medium-sized vegetables or fruits, such as apples, apricots, plums, potatoes or cucumbers). Look at these oranges as if you actually created them. Carefully study how the final product turned out. Look at the shape, size, color, fragrance, surface, weight and all the undulations on the skin. Look at the uniqueness of the "Grand Canyons" (all the dimples) inscribed on each orange's surface.

Do you think, despite their superficial similarity, that all individual oranges are different, unique and special in their own way? Do you think this is true for every fruit, every tree, every human, every life form? Are you missing something by failing to notice this novelty?

Ducks floating in a pond seem like photocopies of each other. In a group, penguins might look identical to each other in shape, size and color. Yet they are all individuals. They have unique personalities, their own families, a different voice, different emotions and varying responsibilities. So do ants, grasshoppers and ladybugs. If you were to adopt two ladybugs as pets, you would more than likely give them two different names. The next time you look at any of these cute creatures, try paying attention to their individuality.

Every one of us is unique and novel in our own way. We have our own stories. Some stories you know; others you don't. If you pay attention to novelty in an individual without looking at him or her as good or bad, you might be fascinated by the variety and richness you see. If you look for novelty, you'll invariably find it. A search for novelty in the ordinary will increase your depth of attention and improve your observation.

☺   **Unique clothes:** Pick your child's (or grandchild's or someone else's) dress. Look for novelty in this dress. See the cute buttons, the color patterns; appreciate the softness of the cloth, the baby fragrance and everything else your senses allow you to perceive. Look at this dress as if you're an expert at designing clothes.

☺   **Sea of novelty:** Look around the house. Find novelty in your toothbrush; see the uniqueness in the apple you eat; find what's special about a flower, even a weed. Look with a fresh, open attitude and willingness to learn when you look at ordinary items in your home, such as the door, windows, microwave, dishwasher, oven, furniture, bed, toothpaste, soap and television. Each of these items has an element of uniqueness and novelty to it. Most of the things in your car, on the road, at work or in restaurants are novel.

Would you agree that you're swimming in a sea of novelty? To appreciate this novelty, you'll have to delay value-based categorizations. This means that you see everything as it is: magical, unique and precious. Even the most mundane object is a product of infinite efforts of the universe and is, therefore, novel and precious. Finding novelty helps you respect and adore the object of your attention. Just like the objects around you and beyond, every individual you meet has a part of him or her that's unique and novel that you can notice, admire and learn from.

☺   **Novelty in individuals:** The next time you meet someone at home or work, pay extra attention to his or her words. Attend to his or her novelty. Ponder the amazing journey he or she may have traveled to be present in your life.

☺ Exercise 2. Use 1 Sensory System at a Time

Pick an apple. Examine it as a two-step process:

1. Hold the apple in your hands and appreciate it as a whole.
2. Now appreciate the apple using your senses, one at a time.

First look at the apple. Attend to its shape, color, stem and all of the marks on it. Maybe there's a sticker describing where it was produced or packaged. Appreciate the uniqueness of this apple. There's probably no other apple in the world that looks identical to this one in every way.

Now engage your sense of touch and feel the apple. Feel its smoothness as well as all of the marks on its surface.

Bring the apple closer to your nose and take a deep breath of its fragrance. Savor this breath for a moment.

Keeping the awareness of the apple in your mind, close your eyes and imagine that the apple is filled with empty space. Imagine this entire space. Imagine the space gradually filling with soothing, white light.

Open your eyes, take the first bite of the apple and close your eyes again. Notice the taste of the apple in your mouth and try to gently suck any juice that comes out of it. Once the juice stops flowing, chew once and again enjoy the taste and suck the juice that is released. Repeat this for a total of five chews. You can finish off the last pieces of this bite and then take the second bite of the fruit, repeating the exercise until the apple is all gone.

Note two specific observations with this exercise.

1. This exercise may have introduced you to the uniqueness of the apple. Now, you may realize that each apple has its own attributes that are unique and precious.
2. You can discover uniqueness more effectively if you use one sense at a time.

You can do this exercise with any other fruit or vegetable you like. Can you appreciate other aspects of your environment using one sense at a time? This approach is excellent for training your attention and bringing it back to the world.

Exercise 3. Find One New Detail (FOND)

Exercises 1 and 2 are excellent to practice in a quiet room by yourself. They also help you deploy your attention where you choose to anytime you find that you are mindless. A practical version of these exercises is the find one new detail (FOND) exercise. In this approach, you pay attention to an object until you're able to find at least one new detail that you didn't know before.

☺   Find four small objects that are familiar to you. If you can't easily find four objects, use the four fingers of your right hand. Straighten these fingers and first study them as a whole and individually. Now try to discern the following four new details about your fingers that you may not have paid attention to previously.

Compare the length of the index and ring fingers; which one is longer? (Hint: It varies from person to person.)

Does the tip of the little finger cross the second joint line of the ring finger? (Hint: It varies from person to person.)

Can you individually fold any of your fingers and touch the surface of your hand while keeping the other three fingers straight? (It may not be possible to do this. Fingers are connected to each other and do not like to move alone.)

Now turn your hand and look at the roots of your nails. Which of your nails have a semilunar white area at the base?

Did you learn a few new details about your fingers with this exercise?

If you picked four familiar objects such as a cellphone, pager, pen and a button on your shirt, find one detail that you did not know before about each object. For example:

What specific words are displayed when you turn on your cellphone?

Do you have seconds displayed with the time in your pager?

Is the make of the pen written in an italicized or a plain font?

What's the color of the buttons on your shirt?

The FOND exercise will make you not only more aware of your world, with familiarity, but also more likely to become fonder of things around you. As a result, you'll learn more, find it easier to decrease the load of your thoughts and possibly have lower stress. The FOND exercise is particularly helpful when you're in a familiar environment. It's another way to make the world around you a bit more interesting. While the exercise is designed for just one new detail, you can try to find as many details as you want to.

Before we go to the next exercise, think about when you can seek novelty, use one sense at a time or find one new detail. Practicing these exercises several times during the day will help train your attention. Two to four times a day is a good goal. Consider attention training the same way you would physical activity.

Exercise 4. Contemplate the Story

So far, each exercise and concept has been directed to bring your attention to the outside world. The exercise discussed next is an exception that's a mix of remaining with the world, yet gingerly entering the mind.

☺ **An apple's journey:** Hold an apple in your hand. Give it a name, say Applina. Become mindful of Applina by attending to her with all your senses one at a time. Now look at Applina and allow yourself to imagine her story. Right from a little insecure blossom on a tree in an orchard, Applina has had a successful career. Take your imagination to the orchard — to the tree, the branch, and the blossom from which Applina started. Imagine the span of time that has elapsed between that time and now. Imagine the space that separates you from that orchard.

The blossom was able to avoid the vagaries of the wind and the rain. It also survived the onslaught of insects and any number of other threats that could have destroyed it. Slowly the fruit evolved from a small, sour baby apple to a fully grown apple of this size. When ripe, Applina was picked, labeled, stored, waxed and then transported — probably from thousands of miles away. In her journey with the other apples, she was sometimes buried and uncomfortable, and at others on the surface and breathing fresh air. Imagine traveling with Applina in her journey. The journey across the country may have given Applina a few marks on her surface.

Finally having arrived at a grocery store, she was evaluated and placed for purchase. Applina wished to be bought before she became old and perished. Fortunately you found value in her and purchased her for the advertised price. She is now ready to fulfill her promise, willing to sacrifice herself for your nourishment.

Every single item around you has such an amazing story that converges to one person: you. Bring your attention to all that surrounds you; pause and think about how each of the things plays a role in your life. Things such as adhesive tape, pencils, pens, paper, a pager, a cellphone, toys, clothes and your car are just some examples. Hundreds of thousands of people may have worked together to bring you these familiar, everyday items. If you can train yourself to think about the story, you may develop a skill to learn a deeper reality and pay greater attention because you have a newfound respect for everything. This skill will also help you avoid rushing to judgments and refine your ability to try to understand others. Such attention makes everything seem special and causes the kindness that's an inherent part of you to bloom. This is a particularly important attribute to carry for your loved ones and friends.

The fact that a particular group of friends and loved ones is a part of your life is a miracle. With the universe so big, and with more than 7 billion of us on this planet, the chance of a particular group of individuals being present in your life is unimaginably small, certainly smaller than winning a big lottery. Every human being connected with you represents a true miracle. Consider every relationship, at home or at work, a true blessing, a gift to treasure.

With your ability to think about others' journeys, you might realize that you encounter most people and things somewhere in the middle of their journeys. You meet your parents, your spouse and your friends in the middle of their lives; you don't know their beginnings and may not know their ends. You know most of the items in your home in the middle of their journeys, not at the beginning and probably also not the end. Only when you pay attention to them and think about their stories as they tell them can you understand their unique preciousness and complete stories. Most of what you own today was someone else's and will belong to someone else after you pass it on. The purpose of knowing this is to realize the transience of most things in your life. This realization will likely help you appreciate everything around you even more. It'll help you become kinder.

Index

People, acceptance of, 120–124
Perception, 28, 35–36
Physical activity, 220, 224–225
Physical resilience, 38
Praise, 64–66, 177–178
Prayer, 166

Random acts of kindness, 113
Regrets, 138–139
Relationships
   common purpose in, 182–184
   connections and, 170
   flexibility in, 179–182
   happiness and, 138–139, 168
   heartfelt, 55–67
   importance of, 138–139
   kind words in, 171–173
   kindness in, 171
   laughing in, 178–179
   listening in, 173–174
   lowered expectations and, 198–199
   meaning and, 138–139
   praising in, 177–178
   prioritizing, 168–170
   rules for apology, 196–198
   rules for saying no, 195–196
   rules of anger, 189–191
   rules of argument, 186–189
   rules of critique, 192–195
   self-kindness and, 184–186
   sharing in, 175–176
Resilience, 37–40
Resiliency Living program, xii, 16, 73–74, 227–229
Ruminations, 20–21

Screen time, decreasing, 217–218
Self-care, 215–216
Self-compassion, 114
Self-defense, 157–158
Self-discovery, 40
Service, 135, 140
Shared purpose, in relationships, 182–184
Sharing, in relationships, 175–176
Situations, acceptance of, 124–130
Sleep, 226
Spiritual resilience, 39
Spirituality
   defined, 141
   higher life principles, 150–151
   meaning and, 149–151
   path creation, 150
   practice of, 141
   understanding, 149
Stress
   defined, 28
   demand-resource imbalance and, 30–31
   good, bad, and ugly, 30, 34
   as ingrained, 24
   lack of control and, 31–32
   lack of meaning and, 32–33
   logical approach to, 34
Stress Management and Resiliency Training (SMART) program, xii, 228
Stressors, 30–34
   capacity to handle, 33
   coping with, 29–36
   defined, 28
   perception of, 35–36
   as source of growth, 35–36

Suffering, 104, 112–113
Surrender, 203–204

10-week program
   attention training, 41–42, 45–79
   emotional resilience cultivation, 42–43, 80–199
   healthy habits, 43–44, 213–229
   mind-body practice, 43, 200–212
   overview of steps, 41–44
Thought-based meditation, 202
Threats, 19–20
Time, 14, 70–71, 128–129, 165
Transform course, xii
Transience, 61–63, 127–128

Unforgiveness, 160, 167

Waking up
   exercise, 50–53
   in focused mode, 48–49, 50
   with gratitude, 48–53
   suggestions and benefits, 50–51
What is this world? question, 136–137
Who am I? question, 134–135
Why am I here? question, 135–136
Wisdom, 203
Work
   compromise and, 147–148
   higher meaning, 148–149
   humility and, 144–147
   meaning at, 143–149
   serving through, 140

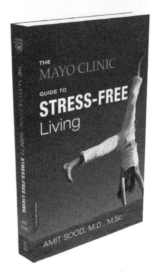